FLAT GUT AFTER 50

5 Simple Ways to Strengthen Your Core,
Prevent Injury, and Look Great
Into Your 60's and Beyond

(SGT.) DOUG SETTER

"As someone who is younger than 50, I found this book to be applicable to me too. The author's details on how and why really helped me understand how important the exercises are. I really enjoyed the chapter on mathematics and health & attractiveness, which provided clear formulas that make sense. I also appreciated how brief and to the point the book was. An easy read!"

—**Lise Cartwright,** author of Mind the Chatter and No Gym Needed

"The breathing, core strength, nutrition and mental re-programming exercises are completely in line with my vibrational teachings and living a healthy life. Doug clearly breathes his topic. Thanks for a terrific book to add to my personal collection and recommend to my clients!"

—**Colleen Wynia,** Reset Your Vibe Energy Coach

"I really, really like this book. Made me train my core more this week. Solid information, scientific studies and good writing.
Very sensible book."

—**Sara Mamykon**

"This book is a comprehensive health with easy to follow movements, including exercises you can do at your desk. It covers steps to better posture and breathing exercises as well as helpful information on good nutrition and improving your gut health. There is a supportive chapter on tools to develop positive reinforcement."

—**Sue Sigourney**

© 2018 by (Sgt.) Doug Setter,
Published by Resilience Press

ISBN–13: 978-0-9878107-6-2
ISBN–10: 0-9878107-6-2

Models: Doug Setter, Lucy Hall, Susan Hyrnchuk, & Monika Kriedmann
Exercise diagrams from Physigraph Clipart (www.physigraphe.com)

DISCLAIMER

Too much too soon is one of the most common reasons for the failure of a new exercise routine. It is also likely to result in injury. Even well-conditioned athletes will experience discomfort or injuries while undergoing new types of training if they push themselves too hard. Remember, the whole aim of fitness training is to enhance life, not shorten it. Fitness is a lifestyle.

Although this book is about fitness, nutrition, and mental conditioning, the author and publisher disclaim responsibility for any adverse effects arising from extreme exercise and dieting and the use of nutritional supplements without appropriate medical supervision.

The intention of this book is not to replace medical advice or to be a substitute for consulting a physician. If you are sick or not medically fit to undergo physical training, you should see a physician before beginning any fitness training. If you are taking prescription medication, you should never change your diet without first consulting your physician, as any dietary change will affect the action of that prescription drug.

CONTENTS

Disclaimer   v

Introduction: The Gut Stops Here   1

Chapter 1 The Mathematics of Health and Attractiveness   3

Chapter 2 Posture to a Flat Gut   7

    Rolling-Like-a-Ball   9

    Torso Raise   12

    The Lunge   13

    Posture and Health   14

Chapter 3 Gut-Busting Breathing Techniques   17

    Beer Gutology Breakthrough   17

    Breathing for Greater Energy   19

    Breathing Exercises   21

Chapter 4 Six-Pack-Carving Tricks of the Trade   25

    Drawing-in-the-Abdomen   25

    Variations   27

    Isometrics   28

    Isometric Stomach Vacuum   29

A Bodybuilder's Secret   30

The Abdominal Routine   20

Leg-overs   **32**

Reverse Crunch (Hip Raise)   **33**

The Crunch   35

Variations   37

Gut-Flattening Activities   38

Advanced Techniques   38

At Your Desk   **40**

Running   42

Skipping   43

Cycling   44

Walking   44

Chapter 5 The Nutrition Training Table   47

Eating for Energy   49

Foods to Avoid   52

White Death   52

White Flour   54

Milk   55

Caffeine, Nicotine, and Alcohol   56

Metabolic Type   56

Fast Burners   57

Slow Burners   59

Mixed Burners   60

Special Diets   61

Cleansing Diets   61

Beating the Food Allergy Bloating   62

Gut-Busting Bacteria   63

Chapter 6 Plumbing Problem Solutions   67

Chapter 7 Mind Management   71

Visualization   73

Affirmations   74

Journaling   78

Reward Reinforcement   79

Behavior Modification Through Punishment   83

Token System   84

Establishing a Routine   86

Delaying Gratification   87

Environment   89

Relapses   91

Chapter 8 Overcoming Flat Gut Roadblocks   95

A Beer Gut Case Study   95

Putting It All Together   96

ABOUT THE AUTHOR   97

APPENDIX A: METABOLIC TYPE TEST   99

APPENDIX B: WORKOUT JOURNAL   103

APPENDIX C: BEHAVIOR-CHANGING CONTRACT   105

REFERENCES   107

*Exercises in bold for easy reference

Introduction
The Gut Stops Here

It took a two-inch incision to convince me just how important core strength is. At 17 years old, when I had my appendix removed (while on a school trip to Japan), I found myself bedridden and next to useless. Yet within three weeks, I was grinding out push-ups, sit-ups, and running in boots on an army reserve course for the rest of the summer. It was the strength of my recovered core muscles that kept me going. Over the next forty years, core power served me well in the military, mountaineering, hiking, martial arts, sports, and even dating.

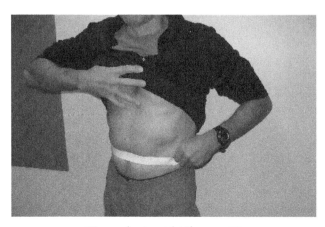

The author's midriff at age 60.

In this short book, I want to share my experiences, methods, shortcuts, and tricks of getting a strong flat stomach so that you, my friend, can take on hard physical challenges, prevent injury, look good and fit well into your sixties and beyond, keep going when others fall behind, or wow the opposite sex and admiring public with a chiseled six-pack set of abs so ripped that you could scrub an oily set of coveralls on them. Or, at the very least, own a strong, flat waistline that you can be proud of.

The beauty of this knowledge is that you do not have to endure torturous exercises and live on carrots and celery sticks. In fact, I am going to show you how posture, breathing, types of exercise, rest, nutrition, elimination, and behavior will carve out a healthy flat gut.

Chapter 1
The Mathematics of Health and Attractiveness

The size of your waist compared to your hips can largely determine longevity and attractiveness. This is known as the waist-to-hips ratio (WHR). To measure your own WHR, measure the narrowest part of your waist (1" above your navel) and divide this number by the widest part of your waist. For example:

1. A man with a 52" waist and 40" hips = 52/40 = WHR of 1.3 (unhealthy)
2. A man with a 34" waist and 34" hips = 34/34 = WHR of 1.0 (healthy)
3. A woman with a 40" waist and 42" hips = 40/42 = WHR of .95 (unhealthy)
4. A woman with a 24" waist and 30" hips = 24/30 = WHR of .80 (healthy)

A healthy woman's WHR is about 0.8, and a healthy man's WHR is about 1.0.

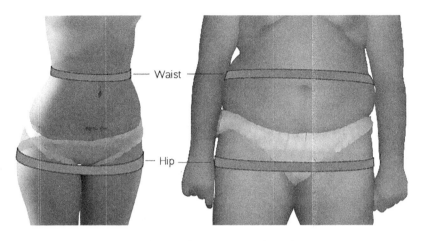

Photographs courtesy of Mikael Haggstrom through Creative Commons

The waist-hip ratio is more important than weight or clothing size. In fact, the WHR, which is the amount of weight that you carry around your waist, can determine future health problems. It is a scientific fact that being fatter around the middle (apple-shaped) is worse than having excess fat around the hips and thighs (pear-shaped). Too high of a waist-hip ratio (WHR) is unhealthy. If you have a wider waist than hips, then you have a higher than normal risk for high blood pressure, heart disease, stroke, diabetes, and even some forms of cancer.[1]

WHR can also determine the attractiveness of a person, especially in the case of women. Most attractive actresses, celebrities, and models have WHR of .67 to .70.

Prime examples are Marilyn Monroe, Celine Dion, Sandra Oh, Sarah Palin, and Kim Kardashian. They all have different weights, heights, body fat, and dress sizes. But the common attractiveness *and health factor* is their waist-to-hips ratio (WHR). Their waists are 70% of their hips. For example, Sandra Oh's 23" waist and 33" hips gives her figure a Waist-to-Hips Ratio of 0.7. Kim Kardashian's 26" waist and 39" hips gives her figure a WHR of 0.67.

This WHR of 0.7 is based on the research of Dr. Devendrah Singh from the University of Texas. Dr. Singh found that 0.7 was consistent in:

1. Many 2,500-year-old Venus sculptures across Europe and Asia
2. All Miss America winners from 1923 to 1987 (0.69 to 0.72)
3. Playboy centerfolds from 1955 to 1965 and 1976 to 1990 (0.68 to 0.71)
4. Across different cultures from Indonesians, Indian laborers, African Americans and Caucasians

Further proving his theory, Dr. Singh also conducted an experiment that measured male brain reactions to silhouettes of women's figures. The silhouettes with 0.7 WHR consistently scored high with 20-year-old male subjects.

Fortunately, attaining the 0.7 WHR does not involve the familiar female fitness philosophy of starvation diets and exhaustive exercise. Hourglass shaping involves correcting muscle imbalance, core strength training, and proper body alignment.

This is to say, a naturally heavier woman with good posture, a well-developed upper body, firm waist, and curvy hips is naturally healthy and attractive. Picture Marilyn Monroe's figure and you have got it. The hourglass shape beats the stick figure in the real world.

The same with the men. A heavy man with a WHR of .85 to .95 with .99 being the most attractive (waist and hips are almost the same measurements) is healthier than a skinnier counterpart with a pot belly. Furthermore, the male with a waist that is narrower than his shoulders or low waist-shoulder ratio (WSR) tends to be more attractive to females.

After instructing hundreds of women in kickboxing, Pilates, and Stomach Flattening, I noticed those who kept training and lasting the longest were the healthier, hourglass-shaped ladies. The hourglass shape had the survivability and durability. The very skinny or heavier women did not seem to last as long.

One of the biggest mistakes that I have researched and observed with women exercising is the tendency to over-train their lower bodies at the expense of their overall figure. This is very common in the middle-aged women who try to diet and train like they did their 20s. Consequently, they end up with tight, flat backsides, tree-trunk thighs, and narrow upper bodies.

The chapters on exercise will address this problem and make recommendations to achieve healthy and attractive physiques for both women and men. Also, a strong abdominal wall minimizes the likelihood of hernias as well as some digestive and back problems. It also goes a long way to being healthier and feeling better.

Chapter 2
Posture to a Flat Gut

Improve your posture, and you improve both your overall body strength and appearance. This is done by strengthening and stretching the right muscle groups so that the body aligns itself automatically. Try this:

Stand up straight. Squeeze your shoulder blades together and pull your neck back in your collar.

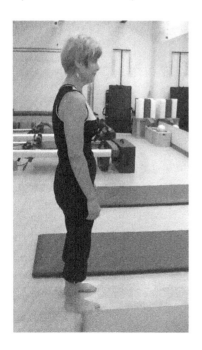 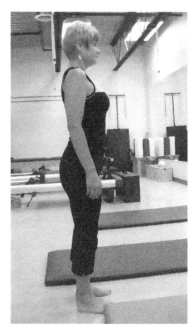

You will probably notice that as your shoulder blades pull together, your chest goes out, and your stomach is drawn inward. This is because the stomach is automatically drawn in when the posture is strong. Most people with good postures naturally have flatter stomachs. The best postures belong to models, dancers, yoga and Pilates practitioners, and most martial artists and athletes. They tend to stand straighter than the rest of the population

One can be physically fit but still lacking strength if your posture is crooked. Consider the wobbly table that you find at some restaurants or coffee shops. You have a hard enough time just steadying your hot drink on a table that tilts to one side. Now think how hard it is to stand on that same table without falling off. The wobbly or tilted table cannot support as much weight as a straight and *aligned* table. The human body is much the same. Even if you are physically fit and gorilla strong, you can appear like a pot-bellied slob if your posture is poor.

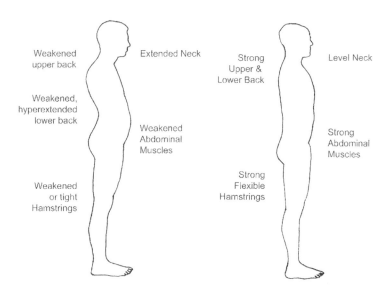

Compare the two postures. The one on the left is typical of most North Americans who spend long hours sitting at a desk, in a car, or slumped in front of a television set. The lower back and hamstrings are tight, and the stomach hangs forward.

Both a sedentary lifestyle AND improper exercise can make the stooped posture worse. For instance, as a young kickboxer, performing hundreds of sit-ups gave me a slumped posture by building up a lump of muscle just under my sternum. It helped protect me against punches and kicks to that area. But it gave me the appearance of a protruding stomach. It was neither attractive nor healthy.

When I trained in classical kung fu with its forms and straight stances, my posture became straighter and stronger. In fact, even with a lay off from lifting weights, I found that I could support more weight when my body was more aligned. Years later, I discovered the body-aligning benefits of Pilates and Ashtanga (power) yoga to relieve my back pain.

Again and again, I have found that posture problems—as well as back pain—can often be solved through **strong abdominal and core muscles and flexible hip flexors and hamstrings.**

Fortunately, we can achieve strong core muscles and flexible hip flexors and hamstrings with a few simple movements borrowed from Pilates and yoga. Namely, Rolling-Like-A-Ball, Torso Raise, and the Lunge.

Rolling-Like-a-Ball

This is a cool exercise for strengthening the abdominals while stretching out the lower back at the same time. It is very effective once you learn how to do it.

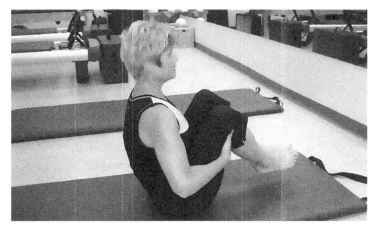

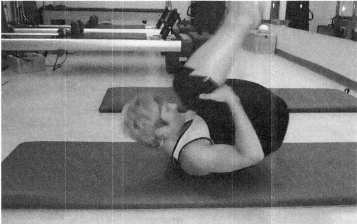

- Start by balancing on your buttocks or your "sit bones." (Your pelvic bones just underneath your gluteus maximus or butt muscles.)
- Place your hands on your hamstrings and hold your body in a tight ball.
- Rock backwards until your shoulders are resting on the mat.
- Then rock forward and shift your hips onto your sit bones, just before your feet touch the mat. Do not let your feet touch the mat.

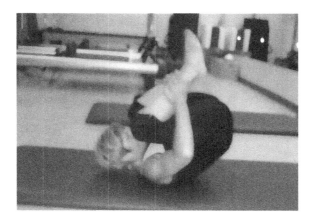

- As you improve, you can move your hands to the outside of your shins and then your ankles.

It took me a few tries to get this exercise right. I initially banged the back of my head and landed flat on my back. The trick to doing this exercise properly is to keep your abdominal muscles tight, like you are holding a quarter in your navel.

Some people are so tight in their lower backs that they require a pad or rolled-up towel (nicknamed a "speed bump") by the small of their backs. As you get used to rolling over this pad, you can systematically unroll the towel until you are rolling like a ball on a flat surface. Do not despair if you do not get this movement on the first try.

I once trained two triathletes who could not do this movement until I placed a rolled-up towel near the small of their backs. Each time they rocked back and forth, I unraveled the towel a little bit. Within a couple of minutes, they were doing the exercise almost perfectly. They had literally retrained their nervous systems to a new movement. So, there was no muscle building or fat burning involved. It was all a matter of reprogramming their bodies to a healthier, stronger state.

Perform 4 to 12 repetitions. The slower the better.

Torso Raise

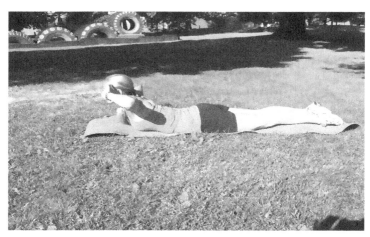

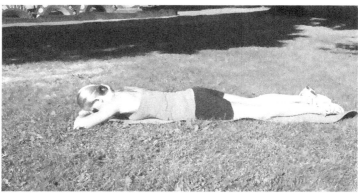

1. Start by lying facedown on your mat with your arms by your sides.
2. Keeping your legs on the mat, raise your head and torso off of the mat. It is important not to hyperextend your chin, which tilts back the neck.
3. Strive to keep your head straight and look at the floor, about a foot to your front.
4. Hold for two seconds and lower slowly.

If you cannot perform a torso raise with your hands on your

forehead, just start out with an easier variation.

Stage 1: Raise just your torso, with forearms on the mat.

Stage 2: Raise your torso with arms by your sides.

Stage 3: Raise your torso with the backs of your hands on your forehead and your elbows wide. When you can perform 12 of these, you can move onto more advanced moves in my book: Strength Endurance Secrets: Build an Unstoppable 2nd Wind.

The Lunge

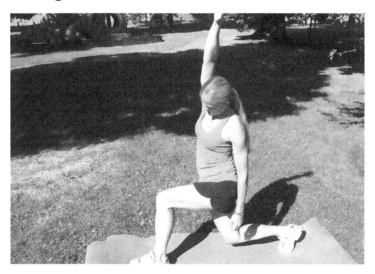

This is a good movement to perform after you have completed abdominal exercises. Step forward so that your front leg (say the left) has the knee lined up above your ankle, but not past your toes. Keeping your rear leg slightly bent or straight (in this case, your right leg), reach straight up with your right arm.

The lunge is very similar to the martial arts stances found in karate (called Zenkutsu Dachi), tae kwon do, and some forms of kung fu. Some forms of the lunge are also found in yoga's warrior postures.

The lunge stretches the hip flexors and strengthens the lower back. This helps realign the pelvis so that it is straight and not hanging forward (as seen in many office workers). A properly aligned pelvis can take away the "pot-belly" appearance from long hours of sitting.

Posture and Health

Walk down any busy street to notice just how many people have improper posture. Office workers, for example, are noticeable for their rounded shoulders and the exaggerated curve of their lower back. This is often the result of long hours of chair sitting. As they sit for extended periods of time, the upper body slouches, the head leans forward, intestines hang below the rib cage, and the hamstrings tighten. To top it off, after eight hours of this kind of abuse, the average desk jockey heads home behind a steering wheel or on a cramped bus. Once home, they flop in front of the television and stare mindlessly at the screen until bedtime. It's a small wonder Western civilization is filled with physical wrecks.

A strong posture allows the human spine to curve naturally. If you were to hang a plumb bob alongside your body, it would run along the ear, the shoulder joint, the hip joint, the middle of the knee, and the ankle bone. To check your own posture, a crude reference point is to stand with your heels, back and head against a wall. With these points in contact with the wall, there should be approximately a hand's thickness of space between the small of your back and the wall.

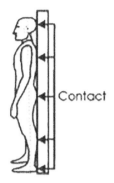 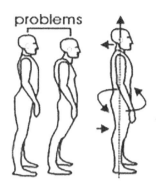

As mentioned previously, most people have the forward head and slouched upper body, otherwise known as Kordosis. Other weakened or misaligned back conditions are the sway back (a kind of a bow-shaped posture), the "duck back" (as seen in many military types with a flat back and protruding butt), and the flat back (with this condition, there is a straight line from the neck down to the legs caused from over-tight hamstrings and back muscles). This last condition is notable because at first glance, the person appears to have no butt and that only one's imagination or a good set of suspenders is holding up their pants.

Posture is much more than cosmetics or dinner-table etiquette. Good posture allows better digestion, circulation, and ease of movement. Posture also reflects the way you present yourself to the world and the way you project your confidence—or lack thereof.

Chapter 3
Gut-Busting Breathing Techniques

Beer Gutology Breakthrough

"It's finally out of the way," my client exclaimed. He was a white-haired, wise-cracking guy in his late 50s.

"What's out of your way?" I asked. "Your attitude?"

"Nah," he replied. "My gut finally shifted out of the way, and now I can keep my leg straight and touch my foot."

Previously, my client had trouble just *seeing* his feet, let alone touching them. We had been working hard at leaning out that personal beer keg of his. While he was fairly strong, he had a heck of a time with flexibility, endurance, and movement.

That is, until he got some control of his breathing.

He was often inhaling and exhaling at the wrong time and holding his breath and panting and gasping like an old steam engine. We finally got him to exhale deeply while performing abdominal exercises. Then with Hindu Squats. Then other exercises.

Part of the problem was that his paunch was pushing against his lungs, especially **while on his back.** It was the pressure on his lungs that made it difficult for him to breathe or concentrate on what he was doing. He jokingly bragged about his "45-pound handicap."

The trick was trying to get him to breathe with a gut that was smothering him. When we tried different angles, like kneeling, on his stomach, and on his side, and really focused on his breathing, he finally felt a "shift" inside his rib cage.

WHEN VERY OVERWEIGHT PEOPLE LIE ON THEIR BACKS, THEY HAVE DIFFICULTY BREATHING DUE TO THEIR STOMACHS PRESSING DOWN ON THEIR LUNGS.

You see, many people's stomachs get bloated from lack of exercise, slouching at a desk, eating junk, and guzzling massive amounts of beer. Not only is there a layer of (cutaneous) fat just under the belly skin, but also (visceral) fat amongst the internal organs. The weight of the internal fat and a weak stomach wall *lets the internal organs sag below the ribcage.* When the gut sags, so does the person's energy.

Our objective is to draw the internal organs back inside the rib cage. The problem with many fitness programs is that they try to flatten a bulging belly with a one-size-fits-all approach of "burning more calories" and lots of cardio exercise. They almost always skip body alignment and the essential breathing techniques. So, the pot-bellied client often gets spindly arms and legs, lower back pain, and still has a large, protruding belly.

With the deep breathing technique, my client, Steve, was able to touch the foot of his extended leg. His agility has also improved to where he can almost stand up from sitting cross-legged *without the use of his hands*. (Watch the video here: https://www.youtube.com/watch?v=YxoHP2p666o)

Instead of being breathless after exercising, he calms his breath in less than a minute. He literally breathed his way to greater strength, flexibility, and a flatter stomach.

Breathing for Greater Energy

Next to a weak posture, a person's breathing pattern is the next dead giveaway to their fitness level. Fit people tend to breathe slower and easier. Unfit people tend to gasp and pant. When you watch animals or children playing, they will run themselves to exhaustion, stop, catch their breath, and then run around some more. The average adult acts terrified of taking in a healthy lungful of air. It is as if they have forgotten how to breathe. This really is a tragedy since when you run out of breath, you run out of performance, period. You can pick out most of the unfit people during an exercise class. They are the ones who are choking and gasping in the back of the room. People with low stamina usually hold their breath or pant when they exercise. Fitter people tend to take longer, calmer breaths. Watch professional athletes in action and you will often see them breathing calmly and deeply.

Controlling my breathing helped me win a welterweight kickboxing championship against a younger, fitter opponent. By the fourth round, he was out of breath—and out of gas—at which point his coach threw in the towel.

Proper breathing increases the absorption of oxygen into the blood. The coordination of breathing with exercise helps relax muscles and release tension, especially in the neck, shoulders, and mid-back. Strong exhalation can draw strength from the deep support muscles. This is why weightlifters and martial artists often yell or shout as they exhale. This allows them to bring muscles into play that they do not normally use.

To make the most of your effort, during most abdominal exercises, breathe out while contracting your abdominals. This will give you deeper contractions and harder, more defined muscles. You will also be getting better results for your efforts than the red-faced beginner who grunts through a basic routine.

To understand what I'm talking about, try the following experiment: take a deep breath and then hold it while performing a crunch[2] or sit-up. Not much fun, is it? Now try letting your breath out as you do a crunch or sit up. It might feel strange, but it should be easier. **Note: It is too much carbon dioxide rather than not enough oxygen that causes fatigue. This is why it is essential to breathe out stale air during exercise.**

Deep breathing is a long-lost ability for most people. With the exception of singers, public speakers, marksmen, martial artists, and some athletes, most people gobble down bits of air mostly through their upper and middle lungs. This restricted breathing uses as little as one-tenth of one's own natural lung capacity![3]

Fortunately, proper breathing and exercise can improve most of these conditions within a few weeks. Most of these breathing exercises can be done at your desk, in your car, or waiting at a bus stop and even with casual practice, the benefits are noticeable.

For those who would like a little more formal breath training, consider the following techniques that can be practiced just about anywhere. However, do not be fooled by the simplicity of these exercises; they are simple, but effective.

Breathing Exercises

1. Take a deep breath and then force all of the air out of your lungs. When you think that you cannot exhale any more, tighten your abdominals and force out a little more air (do this three times). Repeat this exercise three or four times throughout the day with a few hours break in between. At first, it will feel like you are running out of air, and you might start coughing and feel a bit dizzy. If performed correctly, you should feel this deep in the lower abdominals. Usually, it takes about five to ten sessions to learn to do this properly, and then it becomes a habit.

2. Next, repeat the first exercise, but exhale while pressing your lips against your teeth allowing only a small slit for the air to escape. This will force your transverse abdominal muscles to contract. Some yoga textbooks claim that this also helps remove toxins from the blood.[4]

3. The next exercise, called the Complete Breath, is a bit more advanced. First, inhale into your lower lungs (this will make your abdominal wall actually swell a bit). Next, expand your rib cage and lastly, raise your collarbone. By contracting the abdominals,

THEN the rib cage and FINALLY the upper chest, you can achieve a wave-like motion. Although it may feel awkward at first, the Complete Breath can be learned within a week and has been used to treat serious breathing conditions such as asthma.[5] In one variation, asthmatic children are taught this technique by having them lie on their backs with a rubber duck on their stomach. They are then encouraged to perform the Complete Breath by making a wave with their abdominals. If you want to try this at home and are missing a rubber duck, a paperback book will do the trick. Eventually, you will find that you can do this exercise sitting up at your desk or in your car.

If you are still feeling that you cannot get the breathing right, we can solve your problem right here and now by reuniting you with your natural-born ability to breathe deeply with one of two sure-fire methods. The first method is to have you sprint up a hill several times in succession. The second and more immediate method is to have you jump into cold water. Do not be a sissy about this. Jump in there. I guarantee that your heart and lungs will immediately kick into high gear and you will have no trouble whatsoever drawing in long, deep breaths. In fact, you probably will not be thinking of much else except your next lungful of air!

I myself have rediscovered this cold water treatment several times over the years. I first read about it in a book called *Zen Combat* (by Jay Gluck) and later in *Chinese Boxing: Masters and Methods* (by Robert W. Smith). It also comes highly recommended by naturopathic doctors and old-time fitness pioneers like Paul C. Bragg and Jack LaLanne. Champion grappler Matt Furey also advocates cold showers.

Another take on the cold shower is the polar bear swim. For

several years, some friends and I would go polar bear swimming on New Year's Day in Vancouver, Canada. It was always good for a laugh, not to mention the fact that it was a great way to clear a hangover—and, I must add, contrary to popular belief, no one ever got sick from doing it.

For me, there is nothing quite like bringing in the New Year with a plunge into cold water. Also, as masochistic as it might seem to some people, it is also a great way to kick-start the day, and it reminds us in less than a couple of heartbeats about the importance of deep breathing.

By now, I'm sure that most of you have found several excuses not to try this little breathing experiment. "Wait a minute!" you're saying. "I can't believe this guy is telling me to go jump in freezing cold water!" Well, here is where we can separate the doers from the talkers. So, you can either start practicing those breathing exercises right now or, alternatively, go hop into some cold water. It's nice to have options, isn't it?

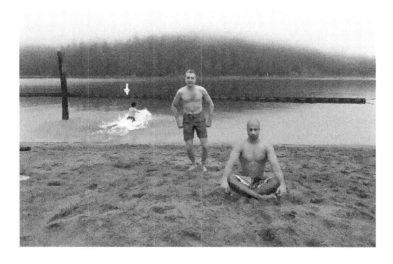

New Year's Day 2018 Polar Bear Swim, Port Moody, BC, Canada, 2018. Me (standing) with yoga instructor Paul Nijar of Yoga Dojo. (Honest, I am having a great time.)

Chapter 4
Six-Pack-Carving Tricks of the Trade

Drawing-in-the-Abdomen

Once you learn drawing-in-the-stomach, you can use this exercise for life, sitting, standing, or lying down. Most males do it instinctively around females—while on the beach, anyway. For those of you who are familiar with yoga, it is basically the same exercise as the hatha yoga asana, Uddiyanna-bandha, and it goes like this:

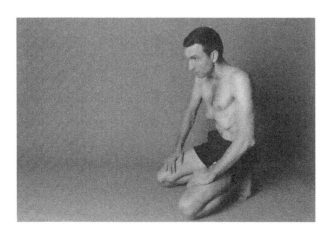

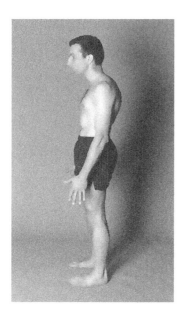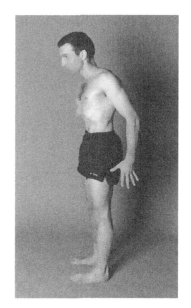

1. As with the first breathing exercise, while standing or sitting upright, take a deep breath and exhale fully.
2. While holding your breath, draw in your stomach (i.e., suck in your gut).
3. Now hold it for a few seconds (try a slow count of ten).
4. Relax and inhale.

You can start out standing, sitting, or kneeling, then later progress to arching your back while pressing down on your thighs. A more advanced technique is to exhale while bending forward at the waist.

Be advised: you should only practice this exercise on an empty stomach. Start out two or three times per day and increase your repetitions gradually. As this movement tones the internal organs, it often causes another kind of movement. So, expect more regular trips to the washroom, as your body might be doing a bit of house cleaning.

You really should stop reading now and do this exercise. It is great. If you want a video demonstration, go to: https://www.youtube.com/watch?v=J9o7lM1UET0

This is a great exercise for the abdominals and internal organs. Once you have mastered this technique, it will stay with you for life, and you can practice it almost anywhere. In fact, you should be able to do it right where you are while reading this book. It really is that simple.

Variations

1. Exhale, hold your breath, and then move the gut in and out several times.
   a. Beginners: 3–4 sets of 10 repetitions
   b. Intermediate: 3–4 sets of 25 repetitions
   c. Advanced: 2 sets of 50 repetitions

A kung fu sifu (instructor) I trained under used to start each class with three sets of 30 repetitions of drawing-in-the-abdomen. We eventually got up to two sets of 50. This instructor was also a heavy beer drinker. Yet through this technique and several breathing exercises, he possessed a rock-hard gut that he let students punch and kick. After a few months of training with just the breathing exercises, punches, and kicks, everyone in the class developed solid midriffs.

2. To exercise the sides of the waist, around the "handles," draw in the gut while pressing lightly with one hand on your thigh and tilting your body to that side.

Isometrics

Isometric exercise was very popular in the 1930s up until the 1970s, when Charles Atlas presented his muscle-building course of "exercise without movement or equipment." I have used it with good results over the years and find isometrics is a good supplement to training.

For instance, if you press your palms together in front of your chest, you are exercising your chest and shoulder muscles isometrically. Ideally, you should keep the pressure up for about 80% exertion for six seconds at a time. There are several variations, but six seconds tends to be the most frequently used.

You can train the abdominal muscles isometrically almost anywhere. That is part of the beauty of isometrics. The following six-second exercises can be performed almost anytime.

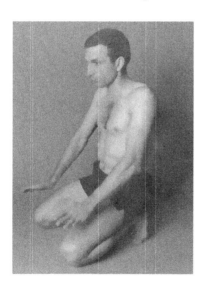 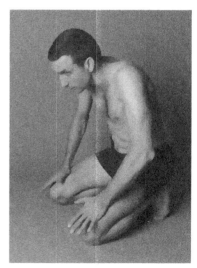

1. While standing, sitting or kneeling, take a deep breath and push down on your thighs. Exhale while you push down and try to bring your rib cage into your hips. After six seconds,

release the pressure and take a few deep breaths. Repeat the exercise a couple more times.

2. Repeat the above while pushing down with one hand on an object (e.g., the window ledge) or a thigh. Relax after six seconds and repeat using the other hand.

3. While sitting, lean back until your stomach feels tight and then twist to one side. Hold for six seconds and then repeat, twisting to the other side.

Isometric Stomach Vacuum

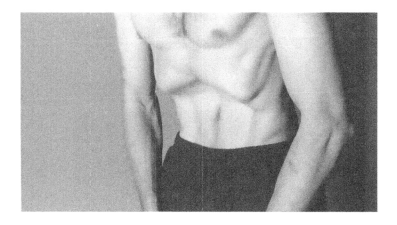

Here is a more advanced movement for **after** you master drawing-in-the-abdomen and the stomach isometrics. First, while sitting, kneeling (easiest), or standing, draw in your abdomen as in the drawing-in-the-abdomen exercise. Then bend over at the waist and push down on your thighs for six seconds. You should notice that a column of muscle sticks out while the sides of your gut draw inward. The first few times, it is likely to feel quite strange and may take some getting used to; however, with regular practice, you can do it almost anywhere.

A Bodybuilder's Secret

In 2002, a friend of mine showed me an abdominal routine that he had learned from bodybuilding legend Shawn Ray. When I first learned the routine, it was thrashing me. I was amazed at how tired I was the first couple of times. But by the fourth session, I could perform three sets of 30 repetitions and had a solid six-pack set of abs that kept me going through kickboxing workouts and hard physical work. And I was only following this routine once per week.

The Abdominal Routine

It is very important to follow this sequence. And if solid stomach muscles are your priority, you should be performing them at the beginning of your workout.

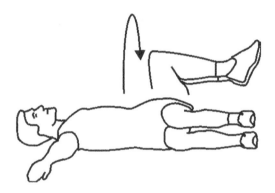

1. First, exercise the abdominal obliques, as these are the body's stabilizers and need to be pre-fatigued.
2. These body stabilizers will tend to assist the other abdominal groups during an abdominal workout. You will want to tire them out so that the other abdominal groups get more

work. Side-to-side movements such as leg-overs will work this area.

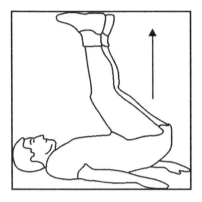

3. Next, work the lower abdominals. As bodybuilders, athletes, and formerly pregnant women can tell you, this is a soft area of the body that is difficult to strengthen. Movements such as leg raises will work this area. Again, you want this area pre-fatigued so that you can really work the next stage.

4. Now, work the crunch for the upper abdominals. With the other abdominal groups already fatigued, the upper abdominals have to take on most of the workload. This is like most of a rowing team suddenly stopping and leaving two members to keep rowing. The upper abdominals get far more work than if they were cruising along with the rest of the abdominal "crew."

For optimum training, there should be no more than three seconds in between exercises. Otherwise, each subsequent group of abdominal muscles will recover and end up "sharing the load" with the other abdominal groups. This means less work and fewer results. It is better to do fewer repetitions with NO rests in between than to perform more repetitions, but have long rests in between sets. The no-rest method means more work for each set of muscle groups, but also superior results in less time.

If you are a beginner, start with one set of 3–5 repetitions of each movement and work your way up to three sets of 20. Then, and only then, should you increase the difficulty of the exercise. Otherwise, you can get burned out and frustrated.

For quick results, try this basic routine three times per week.

Leg-overs

Leg-overs are good for training the obliques. To begin, lie on your back with your arms spread out at right angles to your body. Now, begin to swing your legs from side to side, exhaling each time you swing a leg toward the middle and inhaling as your leg touches the floor on either your left or right side. Work up to 20 repetitions before increasing the difficulty level: lie on your back with one leg straight out on the mat and the other leg toward the ceiling.

Beginner Level: Swing only one leg side to side at a time.

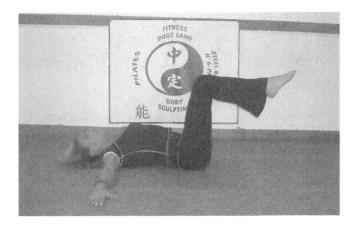

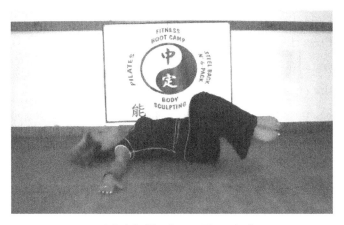

Modeled by Susan Hyrnchuk

Intermediate Level: Bend your knees up to the ceiling and lower both legs over to one side. Touch the floor (no resting) and raise your legs back over to the other side.

Advanced Level: Straighten both legs toward the ceiling. Lower your legs to one side, then to the other.

Reverse Crunch (Hip Raise)

The reverse crunch is a good bet to target the lower abdominals. To begin, lie on your back with your arms by your sides and pressed downward against the mat. Cross your ankles, aim your feet toward the ceiling, and take a healthy breath. As you exhale, raise your hips off the floor and hold the position for a couple of seconds before lowering the hips back down to the mat. For a stiff back and tight hamstrings, you might have to prop up your hips with cushions or a folded mat or lie on an abdominal board with your feet elevated.

For maximum results:

- Press the small of your back into the mat BEFORE you raise your hips off the mat. **This is important, as it will lessen the chance of back injury.**
- Keep tension on your abdominals by NOT resting between movements. Lower your trunk until it just touches the mat and then raise your hips back up again. This way, you get more work done in less time.

Beginner Level: Keep your knees bent (crossing your ankles is optional) and lift your hips so that your tailbone leaves the mat. Slowly lower back to the mat.

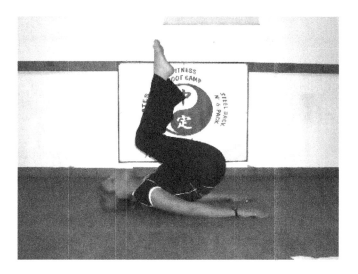

Intermediate Level: Straighten your legs toward the ceiling and raise your hips so that your tailbone clears the floor. Then, slowly lower your hips back to the mat.

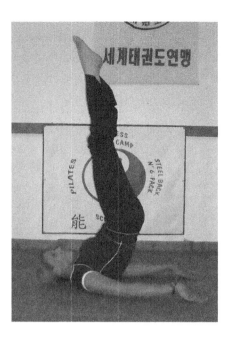

Advanced Level: Point your legs toward the ceiling and arms firmly at your sides, pressing into the mat. Raise your legs, hips, and lower back up to the ceiling and hold for two seconds before lowering your hips to the mat. When you raise your lower body, most of your weight should be on your shoulders and upper back.

The Crunch

Known by many, hated by a few...the crunch is a good, safe method of training the upper abdominals. Start out lying down with your knees bent and feet flat on the mat. There should be about a fist's width of space between your knees. **Press your spine into the mat** and cradle your head or just reach with straight arms and curl your upper body forward until your shoulder blades clear the mat. Exhale on the way up and inhale on the way down.

To really make each movement count:

- Squeeze the abs and exhale fully when you curl forward and up. Imagine that you are trying to crush a basketball between your rib cage and hips.
- DO NOT rest your shoulder blades on the mat between repetitions. Instead, just barely touch the mat and curl up again so as to keep tension on your abs.
- Keep about the width of a fist between your chin and chest to avoid straining your neck.

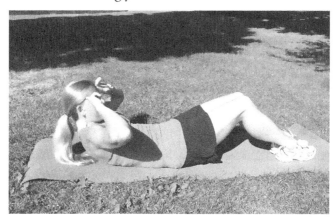

(Note: hands just touch or gently cradle the head.)

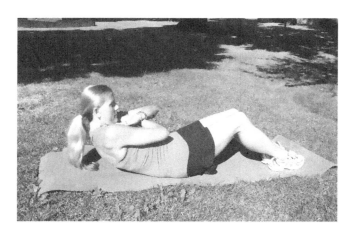

Variations

1. Hold your arms across your chest and raise your shoulder blades off the mat. Perform 20 or more micro-crunches (less than an inch at a time). This is great for ending the abdominal routine.

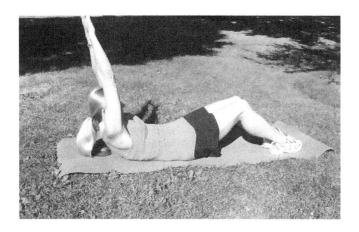

2. While lying on your back with knees raised, look at the tops of your knees and extend your arms while lifting your torso off the mat. As you raise your shoulder blades from the mat, reach for the outside of your knees.

Please remember that even crunches can be futile if they are performed in a sloppy manner. A prime example is a heavyset guy I observed at a gym who was just butchering the crunch exercise. While lying on his back, he would slam his butt into the mat to bring his shoulders up and then ram his shoulder blades back on the mat. He did this while holding a newspaper (that he was attempting to read) up in front of his face. Where is a camera when you need one?

For good results, you have to concentrate on your workouts. Read the paper afterward.

Gut-Flattening Activities

Certain activities will trim that waistline in a subtle fashion without taxing your energy. Walking, running, cycling, ice skating, Rollerblading, gymnastics, most team sports, canoeing, sailing, swimming, dancing, and even gardening engage your abdominal core muscles. Personally, I like the way that many martial arts train the abdominal muscles. For instance, kicking will strengthen the abdominal muscles while stretching and strengthening the hamstrings and lower back. I read about a book editor, Mark Bricklin, who overcame back pain by practicing tae kwon do. I also personally know a tae kwon do instructor who overcame his own back pain by practicing tae kwon do.

Even the simple act of sitting on a stability ball will help strengthen your abdominal muscles.

Find your own favorite gut-flattening activity and stick with it. Just start out gradually and enjoy it.

Advanced Techniques

When you want to test your abdominal and upper-body strength, try the following gymnast positions.

- Cross-Legged L-Seat. Sit on the floor with your legs crossed and raise yourself off of the floor while supporting all your weight on your hands. At first, you might not even be able to move, but after a while, you should be able to clear the ground for a few seconds at a time. Try this three or four times per week until you can hold the position for about ten seconds.

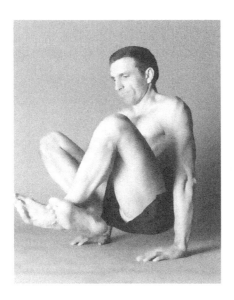

- Basic L-Seat. This is a nice little personal test to check up on your own upper-body strength. To begin, sit with your legs straight out in front of you and arms by your sides with palms flat on the mat. While pushing down with your hands and tightening your abdominals and hip flexors (muscles that raise your legs forward), lift your whole body off the floor. Start out with the legs bent and progress to straight legs. A friend of mine used to do this exercise with a ten-pound dumbbell on his lap.

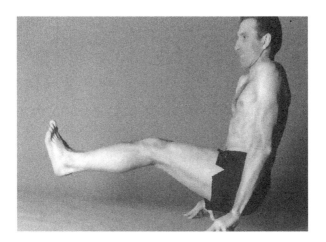

Regular workouts at the gym usually happen only in a perfect world. Since you cannot always make it to your favorite hangout, you sometimes have to look for exercise opportunities wherever you can find them. Your only limitation is your imagination.

At Your Desk

Here are several micro-toners that you can do at your desk. Try these just before a break or when you start to feel sluggish.

1. The Seated Crunch: If you have a reclining-back chair, you can perform this by leaning back as far as you can. Otherwise, you have to scoot up to the edge of your seat before doing the crunches.

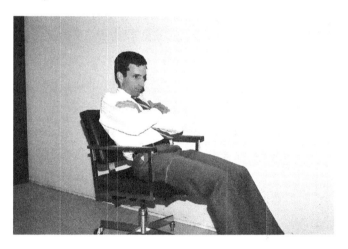

2. Cross Crunch: Lean back in your chair to put some tension on your abdominals. By just alternating the raising of your knee to the opposite elbow, you can work out your lower abdominals and obliques.

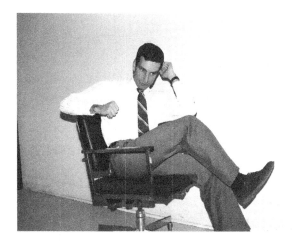

3. Isometric Crunch: While seated, take a deep breath and exhale while pushing down on your thighs or knees. Hold the
position for about six seconds at a time. Ensure that you do
exhale. You can also push down with your forearms to get
more of a deeper crunch.

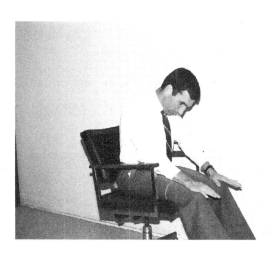

Running

Slow long-distance running is good for conditioning. But sprints engage the obliques (sides of the waist) more. When it comes to sprinting, there are a few different options. One method is to run at a good clip for a set distance, like 100 meters, then jog or walk for 100 meters. Another method is to run hard for a certain time, like one minute, and then jog or walk for one to four minutes. If you are running full-out for one minute, then you need about a four-minute recovery. If you neglect a proper recovery, your speed will suffer.

If you really want to give yourself a good thrashing, try this routine. Begin by running hard for 400 meters or a full minute. Next, do push-ups, squats, or your abdominal routine. Finally, jog for 400 meters and then repeat the sequence three more times. This routine is sure to crank up your metabolism and harden your abdominals. Although you are sure to be sucking wind when you're done, you'll also be waaaaaay ahead of those folks who just shuffle along at a mediocre pace month after month.

There are other ways to optimize your performance as well. If you have the time, run for distance one day and then for speed another day every week. During the rest of the week, go on lighter, easier runs. By following this plan while in the army, I was able to far outdistance the guys who jogged/ran three miles a day every day. They were not working both the slow-twitch and the fast-twitch muscles, so they were not developing the extra power. They were also trotting along at that same happy moderate pace every day, so they were not challenging their bodies to go faster.

If you are planning to run, before you get out there, take the time to ensure that you have good-fitting running shoes and then avoid running on pavement. Running on concrete or pavement is like tapping your heels and spine with a sledgehammer; it is hard on your body, especially your joints. Instead, restrict your runs to rubberized tracks, sand, grass, bark-mulch, or even gravel. It might be wetter and dirtier than pavement, but you will run longer and feel better.

Also, remember to start out gradually. I have known too many people (including yours truly) who have run beyond their capabilities and then spent several weeks recovering from injuries rather than increasing their training gradually. Listen to your body.

Skipping

Skipping is a fantastic physical conditioner. A few minutes of skipping is equivalent to four times the exertion of jogging, and rope jumping will also burn more calories than most other aerobic activities.[6] Best of all, getting started is simple. To find the ideal length of skipping rope for your height, stand on one end of the rope and hold the other end overhead as far as you can comfortably reach. This measurement should give you enough room to skip while you turn the rope. Ideally, one should skip on a wooden floor and wear good running shoes to lessen the shock on the body.

When jumping rope, remember to keep your hands close to your hips as you skip. At first, you may notice that the whole building shakes. However, as you get better, you will develop a steady rhythm and lightness on your feet; as your coordination improves, the skipping gets easier. Start with one-minute sessions twice a week and work up to three times per week. If your ankles get tangled in the rope, just jog or shuffle in place to get your rhythm back before skipping again. When you can skip at around 180 rotations per minute for three 3-minute rounds, consider yourself in fairly good physical condition.

Cycling

Many people in Europe and Asia use bicycles as their primary means of transportation. Here, in North America, there is something embarrassing and even dangerous about pedaling around town on a non-polluting, free-to-park machine. Yet bicycles are a very convenient way to get some exercise in, whether you are shopping, commuting, or out for a relaxing Sunday cycle. The price of a bike can also be less than the cost of driving your car for just one month, and it is a healthy way to physically unwind from the stress of work. As an added benefit, the raising action of your legs cannot help but give the abdominals a workout.

Walking

While it is not a big muscle-builder, walking is highly underrated as an exercise. Walking is a great way to cool down after exercising, a healthy social activity, and the perfect way to end a stressful workday. It is also an easy way to relieve minor injuries, boredom, or fatigue, and a morning walk is a great way to wake up and start the day.

Unfortunately, over the years, I have observed a steady decline in the walking ability of teenagers and young adults. Amongst basic military recruits, more than one-third of all injuries are the result of weak knees and ankles (walking is the best way to strengthen both of these), and while many recruits have athletic ability, most have had little experience walking for extended periods. I find this disappointing, as walking is one of the easiest and most cost-effective ways of maintaining good physical and emotional well-being. In fact, if you live or work in a high-stress environment, consider working a light stroll into your regular routine to mellow out. After all, who ever heard of "walking rage?"

Chapter 5
The Nutrition Training Table

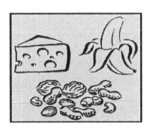

You are a custom-made organism. This means that the diet that works for a pop singer, professional athlete, or someone on a remote island is not necessarily going to work for either a high school student or a middle-aged desk jockey. Just because millions of Northern Asians thrive on brown rice, that does not mean someone from a South American or European background can do the same. The same goes for cabbage, high-protein, low-calorie, or many other diets. Humans have evolved and adapted over thousands of years to the specific conditions and food sources in their region of the world.

Finding the diet that best suits your body's needs can be a challenge. I have seen a wide range of results from people consuming high-protein, vegetarian, and various cleansing diets. Some people thrive on high-protein diets, while others clearly do not. Many times, the dietary needs of your body change over time. Naturopath Dr. Logan Sisk was a strict vegetarian for many years before turning to eating mostly meat. I once read about the Arctic explorer Vilhjalmur Stefansson and his two colleagues who were stranded on floating ice for several months and ate nothing but polar bear and seal.[7] According to the "experts" who follow the national food guides, Stefansson could not have survived.

I have known some vegetarians who were physically fit and strong and others who were weak and sickly. I also once met a fruitarian who was 21 years old. Although she was pretty and had the clear complexion of a 12-year-old, she also had *the build* of a 12-year-old.

When I ate strictly vegetarian, I noticed that I needed less sleep but felt physically weaker. These days, I include some animal protein every day. I also used to eat eggs, half a dozen at a time. Though my cholesterol was always low, I began to get nauseous and feel sluggish. After some experimentation, I found that I feel the most energetic if I only eat eggs a few times per week.

If you are going to follow one kind of diet, it is important to know what you are doing. Take a close look at the people you know who are on the diet already and how their lifestyle relates to your own. Then try the diet for a few days and note the changes in your body and mood. When you become healthier, your body will actually crave certain foods and reject others and you will start eating when you are hungry and not out of boredom.

Eating for Energy

High protein, some fats (fish oils), and high *complex carbohydrate* diets have worked for several of my clients. However, in most cases, if you simply try to eat regularly and stay clear of dairy, wheat, and sugar, you will find that you can keep your energy levels fairly high. Being human, I still have the odd beer, ice cream, or cheesecake. This is why I will talk about guidelines, so that you can have some kind of flexibility and still have a life. That way, too, you don't need to worry about a guilt trip if you occasionally "fall off the wagon." Most people can eat the following:

PROTEINS	FATS	VEGETABLES
Beef	Butter	Green vegetables
Chicken	Almond butter	(broccoli, cabbage, celery, lettuce, Brussels sprouts, etc.)
Turkey	Olive oil	
Fish	Sesame oil	Orange/red vegetables (carrots, yams, beets)
Eggs	Flaxseed oil	Bean sprouts
Tofu	Cashew butter	

GRAINS	FRUITS	MISC.
Brown rice	Apples	"Designer shakes" (protein drinks)
Millet	Apricots	Protein bars
Oatmeal	Pears	
Couscous		
Kasha	Berries	
Kamut		

Please note that just because a food is not on the list, it does not mean that you should exclude it from your diet. This is merely a guideline to nutrient-rich foods. When you eat nutrient-rich foods, such as broccoli or fish, you are saving yourself time and energy. By eating nutrient-rich foods, you are giving yourself a greater energy return than if you eat low-value foods such as doughnuts or cake.

Of course, it is only human to enjoy some junk food occasionally. However, if you pay attention, you will find that the people who argue aggressively about their right to stuff themselves with low-value foods are the same people who tend to be tired, overweight, and/ or generally in a bad mood. While in university, I was told by one professor that "there is no junk food." A registered dietitian (R.D.) also tried to tell me that a bagel was a "nutrient-dense" (packed full of vitamins and minerals) food. Another R.D. recommended cookies and ice cream to *diabetic* children (even the other students thought that she was talking nonsense). The lesson here is that even highly educated people can be biased with information. Some "experts" are paid to say certain things so that they or their university will receive funding. If you are suspicious of any claims, ask people who have had success with whatever the claim is. Quite often, they are very unhealthy and are just repeating the same story sold to them. Rarely do they have any athletic, nutrition, or health background. I have talked to construction workers with a better understanding of nutrition than university graduates.

If you are not satisfied with the foods on the given list, look up other foods in a reputable nutrition book like *Nutrition Almanac*.[8] You might be surprised at what you thought were nutritious foods. For instance, broccoli contains more potassium than bananas, and black currants have over twice the vitamin C as oranges. Also, keep in mind that most organic foods are superior to genetically modified foods. But "organic" food can also be outrageously overpriced.

Try to eat food that is fresh. This ensures the maximum nutrients and the best taste. And while raw foods are superior to cooked foods in many ways, you still have to use some common sense. For instance, grains and many vegetables require cooking to break down the cellulose wall. Although this will result in some vitamin loss due to cooking, keep in mind that there is almost NO nutrient absorption if the grain or cellulose-rich vegetable remains hard and raw. Just try choking down uncooked rice or another grain and you will feel like you swallowed ball bearings.

Some processed foods, such as some prepared camping foods, are actually fairly good for nutrition and taste. Otherwise, highly processed foods tend to lack vitamin C and B vitamins and are also overloaded with harmful substances such as MSG (monosodium glutamate). It serves you well to just eat food as close to its natural state as possible.

Of course, meats and food suspected of spoiling must be cooked to ensure better digestion and to protect against parasites and food poisoning. Eating all raw food all the time, like raw hamburger or even unwashed fruit, runs a risk of food poisoning. Gulping down foods like raw oysters is not the most sanitary habit, either. The oyster does not have much of a filtration system and when you eat the whole thing, you are literally eating its wastes as well. One only has to have a few bouts of vomiting and diarrhea to be suspicious of uncooked food. Ensure that your food is clean, safe, and properly stored. A good rule to live by is: "When in doubt, throw it out."

If you are visiting a new restaurant, it is always a good idea to visit their washroom before eating. If the washroom is clean, then there is a good chance that the food handlers are clean. If the washroom is filthy...well, this is where the food handlers wash up after they use the toilet. Better to appear somewhat rude and leave than risk a bout of stomach cramps and trips to the washroom all night. Besides, a bout of food poisoning will not impress your date, either.

Foods to Avoid

White Death

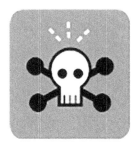

Most sweet substances in nature such as berries and fruit contain vitamins, minerals, bioflavonoids, and fiber. It was primitive people's natural craving for sweets that led them to seek out sources of vitamin C and other nutrients. Unfortunately, this same natural craving draws us to consume sweet, refined substances that lack any food value.

One of the most damaging sweet-tasting substances *over-consumed* in the North American diet is white sugar, also known as sucrose or table sugar. Not only is it highly addictive, but it actually depletes the body of B vitamins, magnesium, chromium, and other minerals. This leads to tooth decay, nervousness, hypoglycemia (low blood sugar), allergies, and mood swings.[9] Depressed people are often suffering from low blood sugar and vitamin B deficiencies.[10] The over-consumption of sugar inhibits the immune system, especially when it is consumed just before sleep.[11]

Refined sugar gives a person a little boost, so they are rewarded with a small burst of energy...however, this burst is followed by a feeling of sudden fatigue. Then, the sugar junkie needs another small fix to keep them going...which results in yet another drop in energy. This is why many people cannot seem to stop eating refined sweets every hour. To top it off, sugar addicts are the most unreasonable people to deal with when it comes to changing their habits.

A couple of simple methods for breaking this sugar fix are to:

1. Keep a journal of your eating habits and then try to figure out when and why you have this addiction. For example, some people eat sugared foods when they are stressed, worried, lonely, or angry.

2. Start eating whole high-fiber or high-protein foods *before* eating any refined sugar. This way, your body will absorb the sugar more slowly than if you just ate the refined food alone. Even eating fiber-rich fruit instead of refined sugar helps satisfy the craving for sweets while slowing down the absorption of sugar.

3. Exclude simple sugars such as fruit juice and replace them with more complex carbohydrates such as whole fruits, grains, and vegetables.

4. Increase your intake of chromium. While not proven to help with weight loss and muscle gain, chromium does stabilize blood glucose (sugar) levels. Chromium can be found in broccoli, cheese, dried beans, chicken, calf liver, and the supplements chromium chloride and chromium picolinate.

Many alcoholics and drug abusers are also hypoglycemic. They constantly crave sweets. Part of the rehabilitation at the Health Recovery Clinic in Minneapolis, Minnesota involves the removal of sugar from the alcoholic's diet. The other offending substance for some alcoholics is wheat.[12] Which brings us to...

White Flour

Bleached wheat flour is easy to store, has a long shelf life, and is easy to work with. It is the main ingredient in bread, pastries, pizza dough, and oh yeah, paste for papier mâché. So, you can image your stomach trying to break down paste. Aside from having next to nothing in terms of nutritional value, white flour actually robs our bodies of nutrition because it impedes the absorption of nutrients from the intestines into the bloodstream. Once it passes through the stomach, the flour forms a glutinous mass that sticks to the sides of your intestines and is difficult to digest. In the old days, eating crackers or dry bread was a common remedy when someone had swallowed a broken chicken bone or other sharp object. This is because it was well known that the gluten would coat the sharp object and often let it pass along without damaging the digestive tract.

As a food, white flour gives you the feeling of being full with little actual nutritional benefit. People who eat a steady diet of this white paste usually have bloated stomachs and thin arms and legs. Most food banks give away bread, pastas, pastries, and other white flour-based products. These items are cheap and plentiful, but hardly the staff of life.

When you are tempted to eat your next doughnut, Danish, croissant, cream puff, or muffin, try eating something with less white flour such as an oat muffin, oatmeal cookie, or date square. By cutting out—or at least minimizing—the amount of white flour you consume, you will be amazed at how much better you feel within just a few days.

Milk

Many people from North European backgrounds can consume massive amounts of milk with no side effects whatsoever. This is especially true if the milk is fresh and unprocessed. A number of famous bodybuilders and athletes have been known to drink gallons of milk and remain physically powerful. At the same time, there are many, many more people whose bodies cannot tolerate the milk sugar, called lactose. This makes most of the population lactose intolerant. Additionally, many people's bodies cannot break down the large milk protein.

Now, before anyone starts protesting about milk and calcium, stop and ask yourself how it is that Native American, Eskimo, Inuit, African, and Asian people were able to lead such vigorous lives BEFORE the introduction of milk. Furthermore, what other animal do you know of that consumes milk (let alone the milk of a different species) after adulthood? The reality is that most humans lose the lactase enzyme after the age of two. Do you think that perhaps nature is trying to tell us something?

Except for some fermented dairy products like cheese, yogurt, and kefir, I have consumed very little milk for the past 25 years. My bones have not shattered, nor have my teeth fallen out. My sinuses are much clearer than they were in my high school years, and I am sick less often.

Of course, it is hard to accept that what you have been force-fed all of your life might actually be poison to you. A simple method to test milk's effects on you is to simply stop drinking it for a week and see what happens. If you have withdrawal symptoms (e.g., runny nose, sore eyes, gas, etc.), you might want to stop drinking it gradually.

Caffeine, Nicotine, and Alcohol

The Western world's three most common drugs are okay in moderation. However, anything more than moderate use acts as a double-edged sword to one's health. On one edge, these three are poisons that pollute the body and overwork the nerves. On the other edge, the stimulants suppress the appetite and are used in place of real food. Consequently, the heavy user gets weaker and weaker while trying to increase their energy by taking more stimulants.

Of course, someone is always arguing about a great-grandfather or great-grandmother who smoked and drank heavily and still lived past 90. Maybe Grandpa did drink a half-gallon of coffee and moonshine and puff on his corncob pipe while plowing ten fields every morning...before breakfast. People like him came from strong genetic backgrounds and worked hard all of their lives. With all that physical activity and a diet that included little or no processed food, they stayed healthy from other aspects of their lifestyle, not *because* of the stimulants.

If you are still not convinced of the harmfulness of excessive tobacco and alcohol use, just pay a visit to skid row in any town or city. There, you get to see close-up the effects of heavy drinking and smoking. Better yet, tour a hospital's cancer ward or the local police station's drunk tank.

Metabolic Type

Just as there are several different blood types among human populations, there are different metabolic types. Determining your basic metabolic type can help you to better understand your body's basic needs in terms of nutrition, exercise, and rest. Fast and slow metabolisms, also known as fast and slow *oxidizers* or *burners,* have been written about for decades.[13] In the book *The Balance*, Oz Garcia[14] describes three basic types of metabolisms. You can take the test in Appendix A to determine whether you are a Fast, Slow or Mixed Burner.

Fast Burners

Fast-burning metabolisms are usually found in hyperactive people who often thrive on anxiety and irritability. They are often impatient Type A personalities who seem to have their adrenal glands stuck on high. They tend to have bursts of energy and have difficulty relaxing. The Fast Burner often has an addictive type of personality and displays obsessive traits or develops an abuse of drugs or even food. Fast Burners may not all be lean and active, but they are constantly looking for quick boosts of energy, usually through quick carbohydrate fixes.

If you are a Fast Burner, you probably skipped the metabolic test and are in a hurry to find answers. Fast Burners, like yours truly, burn out their mineral supplies like there is no tomorrow and have difficulty building muscle. This is why I disagree with diet pills that are mild stimulants that contain substances such as theobromine, caffeine, and ephedrine. These "quick fixes" will only tire you out in the long run.

A Fast Burner must maintain a steady flow of energy from their food. Take a typical eating pattern:

Breakfast: Coffee, toast, fruit

Snack: Coffee or pop and a donut

Snack: Coffee, muffin or donut
Lunch: Juice, yogurt, salad with dressing, bagel
Snack: Diet Coke
Supper: Chicken breast, boiled potato, and frozen mixed vegetables
Snack: Apple

It is painfully obvious that this eating pattern is packed with sugar at regular intervals. While it might fit the low-calorie, low-fat format, it is going to give the eater more ups and downs than a runaway roller coaster.

An effective Fast Burner eating plan would be more like this:
Breakfast: Water, oatmeal, three egg whites
Snack: Peanut butter on whole-grain crackers or chicken fingers
Lunch: Chicken or salmon salad
Snack: Protein shake
Dinner: Water, lean beef, stir-fried or steamed vegetables
Snack: Water, slice of turkey breast

The Fast Burner can tolerate higher amounts of fat and oil, as they need the gradual release of their concentrated energy. Most fruits and fruit juices are high in fruit sugar (fructose) and should be avoided. However, vitamin-rich fruits such as apples, pears, apricots, and all types of berries are okay.

When I find six small meals a day a nuisance, I try to have at least two good sit-down meals per day. I often did this while I was in the military, working around the base. I found that I could actually make faster muscle gains by eating fewer meals but eating those meals slowly.

Those high-speed, Type A people who are too busy to eat must discipline themselves to either prepare their meals in advance (and use plastic containers) or arrange to have two relaxing, uninterrupted meals per day. Many Europeans, like the Germans, eat like this. They have tea and some heavy bread in the morning, a huge (often two-hour) lunch, and then a moderate supper in the evening. If you have been to Germany, you might have been amazed as I was to see stores close, restaurants fill up, and so many people just relaxing during one of North America's most frantic times of the day. Some might argue that this is a slack attitude. However, from my experience there, I would have to challenge anyone who questioned the productivity or good health of Germany's people.

If you are a very active Fast Burner, such as a competitive athlete, you can add more complex carbohydrates, like rice, yams, or potatoes to your diet. As for exercise, Fast Burners often benefit from anaerobic exercise, such as weight lifting, sprinting, team sports, or even yoga. The short duration exercises help build muscle tissue and can have a more calming effect than aerobic exercise.

Slow Burners

On the other metabolic extreme, Slow Burners tend to be easygoing, have low blood pressure and good digestion, and often dislike exercise.

A typical Slow Burner eating pattern is as follows:
Breakfast: Two waffles with butter and maple syrup, two cups of coffee
Snack: Apple
Lunch: Baked potato, egg salad, roll with butter, fruit cup, coffee
Dinner: Salad with dressing, rice, brownie with vanilla ice cream

By now, you can see the low food value and high sugar content of most of these foods. This Slow Burner's energy is going to drop about an hour after every meal. Unfortunately, many of us have grown to accept that afternoon "dinner drunk" syndrome as normal. When you eat properly, you can often go back to work feeling satisfied and alert. An effective Slow Burner eating plan would be more like this:

Breakfast: Two eggs, poached or over-easy, steamed vegetables, one cup of herbal tea

Snack: Protein shake

Lunch: Salmon salad with greens, tomatoes, olive oil and lemon juice, one pear

Snack: Low-fat yogurt or cheese (if you can tolerate dairy) or almond butter and rice crackers

Dinner: Chicken breast and stir-fried vegetables

Slow Burners should minimize their fats and oils and stick to whole fruits such as apples, bananas, and citrus fruits. Bananas and citrus fruits are high in potassium, which is a mineral that tends to be low in most Slow Burners. Grapefruits have been used for decades for weight loss, as they tend to help kick-start a slow metabolism. Be aware that some people are allergic to citrus fruits and might react adversely to them.

Mixed Burners

Only about ten percent or less of the population is estimated to be Mixed Burners.[15] If you are one of these, you will have a fairly even flow of energy unless you "fall off of the wagon" from a steady intake of processed foods, coffee, and reckless living. However, a Mixed

Burner metabolism is not a free ride.

You can take food choices from the other types of burners and determine what works best for you. Sometimes you might perform more like a Fast Burner, and others you might perform like a Slow Burner. You have to find out for yourself.

As for exercise, use anaerobic exercise like weight lifting to slow yourself down and aerobics like running to speed up your metabolism.

Special Diets

There are always new and better diets out on the market. Some, actually work...for a while, but they are difficult to maintain over a lifetime. If you look through an old bookstore or at the library, you will find that many of the "new" diets are simply rewritten old diets. For instance, there was a high-protein diet described in *The Letter of Corpulence* by William Banting written back in 1864.[16] Since then, there have been many duplicates of this concept, like Dr. Herman Tarnowner's Scarsdale Diet or The Atkins Diet. While many of these concepts work great in theory for some people, few of them work for everyone all of the time. In the end, you have to find out on your own what works for you.

Cleansing Diets

On occasion, I go on a cleansing diet for a couple of days. This diet consists mostly of vegetable juices, soups, and some fruits. I couple this kind of diet with regular saunas. After a few weeks of doing this every weekend or every other weekend, I often experience better sleep, clearer skin, and better digestion. These short mono-diets and mild fasts can be beneficial if *they are coupled with lots of rest.* During my younger years, I tried to fast while maintaining a regimen that included hard physical work. It left me feeling like a zombie. Therefore, I can only recommend cleansing diets if you are resting and getting the extra sleep necessary. Body cleaning, like house-cleaning, takes energy to do properly. Long fasts without trained health care supervision can be damaging to your health.[17]

Beating the Food Allergy Bloating

This is a fascinating area. Certain foods can cause problems such as intestinal problems, like Irritable Bowel Syndrome; hay fever; attention disorders; bloating; and even alcohol cravings.

At an early age, I was constantly plagued by sore eyes, nasal drip (runny nose), gas, sleeplessness, and sneezing. I was constantly coughing and blowing my nose, and I went through school with pockets full of tissues. It took me until age 20 to realize that dairy and wheat products were aggravating my hay fever and interfering with my breathing and my ability to gain muscle.

Typical symptoms of a food allergy are dark circles under the eyes (shiners), sore eyes, runny nose, fatigue, drowsiness, anger, shortened temper, and accelerated pulse. These reactions may take effect anywhere from several minutes to several hours after consuming the allergen. This can be a real problem if you have been eating allergic foods all of your life and have simply learned to accept the conditions associated with them.

So, how can you tell if you are allergic to a food? If the offending food is new to you, the allergic reactions will tend to occur almost immediately. However, if the food has been consumed since childhood, you will likely experience a bit of a *coffee-like boost right after consumption*. This will be followed by a drop in your energy level, followed by more cravings.

To test yourself for food allergies, try avoiding each suspect food separately for about a week at a time. What is interesting is that *you will tend to crave the very foods that you are allergic to*.[18] Removing these foods from your diet can be like an alcoholic trying to avoid alcohol. As your body cleans itself of the allergic food, it will experience some withdrawal symptoms, including intense cravings. This is normal. Usually, you can keep the cravings subdued by having a small amount of the offending food. Although the process of removing allergic foods from your diet might take some time to accomplish, it is well worth the effort for the result of feeling better and actually being healthier.

Gut-Busting Bacteria

You can also improve your digestion and waistline by consuming gut-friendly bacteria. This is nothing new, as many cultures have been doing this for centuries, long before the introduction to sterile and highly processed foods. After all, we coexist with trillions of microorganisms that depend on us, as we depend on them. Over the past thousands (even millions) of years, we have worked out an interesting coexistence.

As strange as it sounds, friendly intestinal bacteria actually help us by:
- Improving our immune systems
- Preventing harmful bacteria from infecting us

- Providing vitamins
- Breaking down and helping us absorb food

Outside of exercise and dieting, some types of bacteria can actually change your weight. Biologist Jeffery Gordon[19] and graduating student Peter Turnbaugh from Washington University in St. Louis studied both obese and thin mice and humans. They found that:

- Obese mice and humans had large numbers of a bacterial phyla or division known as Firmicutes and low numbers of another phyla of bacteria called Bacteroidetes.
- Thin mice and thin humans had high numbers of Bacteroidetes and low numbers of Firmicutes.

Then the researchers transferred these different gut bacteria from obese and lean mice into mice raised in a sterile environment. The sterile environment (gnotobiotic) mice soon became fat or thin depending on which kind of bacteria they received from the other mice.

Gordon and Turnbaugh then transferred human gut bacteria into other gnotobiotic mice and fed the mice a typical North American high-fat, high-sugar diet.

Within only 24 hours of receiving these "human" foods, the types of bacteria reversed within the mice. The mice with the fat-human-gut bacteria grew fatter than their siblings. So, more Firmicutes than Bacteroidetes.

This might explain why we sometimes get these crazy cravings like we are driven by some kind of alien force. The evil Firmicute bacteria could be screaming for more fat and sugar while a healthy intestinal tract craves Bacteroidete-friendly food.

The type of intestinal bacteria can also affect your brain. Nerve pulses are constantly signaling your digestive system and brain. This is why we get "gut reactions" and "butterflies in the stomach."

You might know that serotonin, which influences mood, sleep, depression, and aggression, *is more concentrated in the gut than in the brain*. Something like 5%–10% is stored in the brain, and the remaining 90%–95% is in your intestines. So, antidepressants are not going to help your brain very much if your gut is in turmoil. The healthy digestive tract promotes a happy brain.

A study at the University of Toronto School of Medicine and Department of Nutritional Sciences tried an experiment with beneficial bacteria on humans with Chronic Fatigue Syndrome (CFS). The type of bacteria used was lactobacillus, which is found in yogurt.

After two months, the people taking the Lcs probiotics showed a marked decrease in anxiety, including better sleep and less dizziness, fewer appetite changes, and less shortness of breath.

A similar experiment found that the probiotic Bifidobacterium reduced anxiety behavior in mice.

Look at some of the fermented foods consumed by healthy, lean, and reasonably sane cultures. The Japanese natto (fermented soybean), the Korean kimchi, the European sauerkraut, and European and Mongolian yogurt or kefir. Even Captain Cook fed his sailors sauerkraut and saw a significant drop in scurvy.

Here are a few things that you can do to get the benefits of brain-enhancing, fat-reducing intestinal flora:

1. Reduce all white sugar. This means even artificial sweeteners. A 2008 study at Duke University found that rats fed

Splenda had a significant reduction of good bacteria in their digestive tracts.

2. Eat fermented foods. They are good-tasting and cheap. Many ethnic stores have kimchi, Japanese natto, East Indian Dahi, and sauerkraut and are much cheaper than the main supermarkets. Learn to make your own.

3. Avoid sweeteners. This means eat only plain yogurt or kefir.

4. Use probiotics. I find that the greens-type of probiotics work well for me. (I have no commercial connection with any of the brand names.)

Get your intestinal bacteria upgraded and in shape to help your body do the same.

Chapter 6
Plumbing Problem Solutions

Although few people want to hear about a bunch of (bleep) in their intestines, what they may not realize is that if their plumbing is backed up, they are going to both look and feel ill. This is because the colon (large intestine) not only disposes of waste matter for the body (and the bacteria that accompanies it), but it also absorbs vital nutrients from the digested food that passes through it. A blocked colon cannot absorb nutrients efficiently because there is simply too much fecal matter in the intestines. Until it is dealt with, this will inhibit the absorption of nutrients and keep a person ill. While some people might argue that this bloating of the colon is just a few extra calories, one might also argue that these people are literally full of you-know-what. One of my fitness students insisted that his bloated stomach was "hard," and I suppose if you consider a water balloon hard, then maybe it was.

One of the primary jobs of the colon is to remove excess water from digested matter and compress the resulting waste for removal. Without enough water and fiber in your diet, this waste stops moving, and the unpleasant result (as you may have experienced for yourself) is constipation. If you don't know, fiber is the substance that is not digested or absorbed during the first stage of digestion in the small intestine. Because it is not broken down, as the fiber moves on its way toward the colon, it tends to absorb water and actually sweep out the intestines. Bran, fruits, and vegetables provide good amounts of fiber.

Lack of exercise, dehydration, and processed foods are the main causes for constipation, and even some "instant" foods can cause problems in the large intestine. This is the great folly of protein powders, as many of them will actually block up the colon. I found this out the hard way as a teenager trying to gain weight. Instead of huge muscles (like the bodybuilder on the front of the container), I ended up with sinus congestion, a skin rash, and some very unpopular flatulence.

Just as some people can tolerate certain foods better than others, so it is with protein powders. What works for a popular bodybuilder might not work for the average mortal. It is in your best interest to ask around or try small amounts of certain brands of protein powders before investing in large buckets of the stuff.

Keeping the colon clean and happy is very important for overall health. When the body's exhaust system is not working, the toxins start backing up into both the bloodstream and the lymphatic system. As a result, you end up with problems such as sinus congestion, headaches, allergies, acne, etc. The fact is, the body needs to eliminate, and one trip to the toilet every three days is not enough. If you suffer from constipation, you might consider some alternative treatments. Massage, enemas, colonics, herbal therapy, proper eating, and of course, exercise can get you moving and feeling better within a few weeks. Although over-the-counter laxatives may be readily available, in my mind, most are a risky shortcut, as they can irritate the bowels and deplete the body of nutrients. However, if you do need a laxative, the formulae with psyllium seeds are quite reliable, as the ground seeds are high in fiber and expand to absorb a lot of water. Of course, for this reason, be sure to drink plenty of water when you use them.

Through the use of colonics, herbs, massage, and proper foods, you can actually cure yourself of acne, allergies, colds, sore throats, headaches, and fatigue. Removing white flour and sugar from your diet will greatly speed up your stomach-flattening process. Forget the arguments about how much white bread your 104-year-old great-aunt ate or being afraid of hurting the local baker's feelings. White flour plugs up the colon, period. Colon health might sound gross to some people. But it is worth the time and effort to do some internal housecleaning, and you will definitely feel better for it.

Chapter 7
Mind Management

"We are what we repeatedly do. Excellence, then, is not an act, but a habit." —Aristotle

Habits and results go hand in hand. This I can tell you based on my own experience and from firsthand experience with others. While in the military, we had little privacy, and there was no hiding each other's personal habits. We worked, ate, slept, washed, etc. in close proximity to our fellow soldiers. It was never a surprise that the partygoers were often flat broke before anyone else. Or that the guys who dressed and spoke well had plenty of dates. Or that the men and women who exercised frequently had more stamina and were in better physical shape than everyone else. The truth is—with soldiers as well as with all of us—in the areas of their lives where we put the most energy in, that's where we got the most results. There was no hiding that fact, and in the end, it was never about "big efforts," either; just everyday habits practiced day in and day out.

The other thing that I noticed in the military was that people had different motivations for exercising or staying fit. The soldiers I knew personally also had different reasons for staying fit. Some wanted to take physically demanding training, like the paratroopers or pathfinders. Some liked morning runs, while others did it out of necessity. Some were crazy about sports. One guy tried to go AWOL so he would not miss his floor hockey game. Still others just liked socializing at the gym.

Everyone has different motivators toward or away from exercising. Some children learn at an early age to link exercise with either satisfaction or disappointment, depending on their experience. For some, participation in physical activities such as sports means approval from parents, teachers, and peers. This is especially true in high school, where athletes often receive extra attention and special privileges. The story is quite different, however, for those who were physically awkward as children. Often ridiculed while playing sports, bullied by their more athletic peers, or humiliated by gym teachers, these children learned to hate anything related to physical education.

Now in adulthood, some people still feel certain resentments toward structured exercise. Some get their exercise by pursuing the social "singles scene" that is prevalent in fitness clubs. Many overstressed people, like the newly divorced, use exercise as a release to vent their frustrations. Others need the open spaces and freedom of outdoor activities like hiking, skiing, or scuba diving. Still others trudge along, treating exercise as a bitter pill that they have to swallow, or if they can, avoid altogether. It is this latter group that has to find a way to make physical activity a pleasant habit and lifestyle.

There are several psychological methods for changing a lifestyle. Find a method or combination of methods that suits you and stick with it for *at least 30 days*. You will be amazed at the phenomenal results from just a few subtle changes.

Visualization

Visualization is simple, yet not easy. By regularly thinking about or picturing something, you will tend to move toward what you dwell on. Either that, or the object or situation will be drawn to you. Usually, people do not get what they hope for because they are *thinking about several other conflicting things*. They tend to use visualization in a negative way. It is like people actually praying for something that they want and then ending their session with the thought, "but it's not going to happen." Or they focus on what they are afraid of. How many times have you heard, "I was afraid that would happen"?

Even if you are afraid of something else happening, you must keep focusing on your objective and stay positive in your visualizations. You have to look past the obstacles and keep on track with what is important to you. It is like the advice for new drivers, "Keep your eyes on the road, not the ditch." When I was trying out for the Canadian Airborne Regiment, I kept seeing myself wearing the paratrooper's maroon beret. Despite disapproval from some supervisors and peers, I eventually got there. I used the same technique to run marathons, win kickboxing matches, and complete a university degree. Whenever I was not focused on my goal, I often fell short or failed.

Some high performers, like top athletes and entertainers, visualize their success in fine detail. For instance, a rock climber might picture himself on a cliff face. He is so tuned in to the visualization that he can feel the cold or heat of the rock as he moves himself along, from one gripping point to the next. To complete the visualization, he might imagine himself up close, making all the right climbing moves to get to the top and conquer the cliff.

Some people find that it makes the visualization process easier if they put up pictures of the goal they are working toward (images of high-performance athletes, models, vacation spots, vehicles, or houses). When they see these pictures, they tend to think about what they want and subconsciously invent ways of achieving their goals. I used to pin up photos of famous athletes that I aspired to be like. This is why a training environment is important. At the Canadian Airborne Centre, there were chin-up bars and training apparatus everywhere. Most of the walls were covered with flags, graduation plaques, and motivational signs such as this: "Pain means that you are still alive." As we trained, we focused on passing, not failing, and most of us ended up wearing the paratrooper's jump wings.

Affirmations

Aside from picturing what we want, we can also support our mental process by verbalizing and writing down what we want. It's true that what we focus on is what we get. So, if you keep talking about how good business is or how much life sucks, eventually it becomes a self-fulfilling prophecy because you will look for or attract elements that support what you believe. For myself, I have found that just repeating phrases like, "I can do this" over and over can help accomplish certain things when doubt has crept into the back of my mind.

Verbalizing your goals is a very useful tool provided that you:

1. Keep it simple. "Fifty crunches is an easy goal."
2. Keep it positive. "I am getting stronger every day," rather than "I am NOT getting weaker" or "I am NOT a blob."
3. Keep it in the present. Dwelling on the past or "someday" isn't going to work. Goals require action now and they require deadlines.

Obviously, if you keep repeating something that you know is not true, you will not get much in the way of results. This is where writing out the idea or goal will help. However, this does not mean mindlessly writing out the statement over and over, like a grade school punishment. One way to find an affirmation that you can work with is to make two columns on a sheet of paper with the statement (or affirmation) column on the left taking up two-thirds of the page, and the response column taking up the remaining one-third of the page on the right.

Now, write a statement that you expect to be true on the statement side of the page and then write the first thing that pops into your mind on the response side of the page. At this point, it is not uncommon to find some very negative responses dredged up from your past, but don't let this slow you down. You have simply reached the turning point where part of your mind is struggling to hold on to negative thoughts. Be prepared to face the thoughts, accept them, and continue with your affirmations. This may be very uncomfortable at first, but there is no reason to panic. Whenever a protest pops up (e.g., *you can't do this, you are too old, young, weak,* etc.) just thank yourself for the response and keep moving.

We are doing a bit of mental housecleaning here, so don't be surprised if you find more than just dust bunnies in some of those dark corners. Just remember, though, that things that hide in the dark and cast big shadows aren't nearly so scary when we pull them out into the light.

To make your affirmations even more effective, try writing your statements in the first, second, and finally, the third person. Write out the affirmation five times for each viewpoint and try to write these out three times per day.[20]

For example:

STATEMENT / RESPONSE
(First Person)
Working out is easy for me. / What, are you nuts?
Working out is easy for me. / Yeah, and there's no time for anything else.
Working out is easy for me. / And be anorexic.
Working out is easy for me. / ????
Working out is easy for me. / Not you, geek...

(Second Person)
Doug, working out is easy for you. / Says who?
...etc.

(Third Person)
Working out is easy for Doug. / Sometimes.
...etc.

Usually, while writing these statements, there will be some strong protests. After all, most of us were told from an early age that we had certain limitations (e.g., *You'll never do that, Kids today are so lazy, Life is hard...then you die.*). But after a few days, the resistance should begin to crack, with responses like, "Well, usually working out is hard, but sometimes it's easy—like last Wednesday, when I ran for ten minutes without stopping." This is the point where your mind starts to give up some of those old negative beliefs and replace them with more positive ones that are based on recent experience. Of course, not every affirmation will be the same. In some cases, you may find that you are facing weeks and weeks of steady resistance. If there is real resistance to a statement, try letting it go for a while and come back to it later. In the meantime, try a different affirmation.

One of the more difficult statements to deal with has been: "People want me to succeed." Try that one out for size. It is really amazing the amount of trouble or number of problems that most people have with writing out that particular phrase.

More popular affirming statements are:
I am good to my body and my body is good to me.
I am stronger every day.
I eat what is best for me.
I appreciate myself.
People want me to succeed.
Money flows to me freely and easily.

Having said all of that about affirmations, remember that not every method works the same for every individual. If you find that writing out these affirmations is too weird, awkward, or unscientific for you, then please try something else.

Journaling

Many days, you will feel like there is NO progress at all taking place. When you get in better physical condition, you will usually not recognize the subtle changes until you look at previous photographs or measurements, try on old clothes, or hear feedback from friends. This is where journaling comes in, as it is far easier to *stay on track* if you can *keep track*.

To start journaling, you must figure out where you are now. By determining your starting point or **baseline**, you give yourself a reference point. Your baseline can be made of beginning body measurements, time to run a certain distance, number of exercise repetitions, or even time spent on an activity like running, swimming, or cycling. A very practical method is to take your waist-hip ratio (WHR) as mentioned in Chapter 1.

To get somewhere, you must start somewhere. Even if you only walk around the block or visit a gym once a week, that is okay. Just record it.

Even the simple act of riding a bicycle to the store a few times each week is worth recording. By writing down your activities, you become more aware of what you are doing or not doing. I do this with training, writing, and studying. It only takes a couple of minutes per day to mark it on a calendar or make an entry in a notebook. Keep the journal accessible so that you have a constant reminder of what you want to accomplish. You might find, too, that you want to change your goals from time to time. This is important, as it helps to redefine what you want and keep you pointed in the right direction (maybe you don't want a 24-inch waist, after all; maybe you just want a date).

During days of unusually low or unusually high performance, you should mark down what was happening that *week*. This way, you can determine what might be helping or hurting your performance. Changes in eating, working, sleeping, and your personal life will often reflect your training. For instance, if you are excessively tired on Wednesdays after working late on Tuesdays, then you should consider making Wednesday an easy training day or get more sleep on Monday night. Some people insist that they get better workouts early in the morning, especially if their jobs entail standing all day. A bit of planning can bring big results. See Appendix B for an example of a quick and easy training record.

A friend of mine, Mike Feuntespina, is a former international cyclist. He is constantly measuring his performance in martial arts, cycling, or business. He looks for subtle changes in skills and strives to improve them, even if in small amounts. He watches his training like a broker at the stock market, and his performance speaks for itself.

Reward Reinforcement

Maintaining reward systems or positive reinforcement is an important part of building lifelong habits. As human animals, we generally like to repeat the things that we have been rewarded for. The basis of positive reinforcement or habit-changing is that when someone does something and is positively reinforced *immediately*, they will tend to do the same thing again in a similar situation.[21] You will note the word *immediate*. The person who plans to train and diet all year and then reward themselves with a summer vacation has less chance of success than someone who gives themselves *small, but immediate* rewards for training and dieting throughout the year.

The first big mistake that people make with the reward system is *delayed rewards*. Trying to get in shape for a vacation or the forthcoming summer season when it is still several months away might be a good reason to train, but it fails to motivate as a strong reward. To grudgingly drag oneself down to an unfriendly gym or pedal on an exercise bike in the corner of one's basement is just plain punishment. I recall my stepfather recovering from a heart attack by pedaling on an exercise bike. He lasted about two and a half weeks before resuming his usual routine of television-watching, chain-smoking, and beer-guzzling after work. His second heart attack followed a few months later, at age 46. The problem was that there was no reward linked with the daily activity. Unfortunately, there was also a hell of a punishment waiting for him as a result of his slipping back into old habits.

Frank, who is a retiree, used a more successful method of behavior modification.

After failing several times at exercising, Frank put exercise into his own established routine. This original routine was coming home, grabbing a beer, and sitting in front of the television. What Frank did was come home, put on his sneakers, walk around the outside of his house once (the behavior), and then have a beer (reward). After a few days, he was walking around his house several times before sitting down to a beer. Gradually, Frank set goals of greater distances before accepting his reward. He must have really wanted that beer, as he was soon jogging a quarter mile every day.[22]

I cannot stress enough the importance of immediate rewards during a habit-changing program. The shorter the time span between the activity and the reward, the stronger the habit-forming bond. It is even better if you can incorporate the reward into the activity. For instance, many of my own workouts involve going to a good gym, talking to interesting people, listening to good music, and sometimes, eating at a restaurant with friends after the workout. For me, this is a great reward for working out, and I associate my experience at the gym with good times and good folk. However, suppose that I was in total pain throughout my workout, the people in the gym were all rude and unwashed, my locker was broken into, and the restaurant food that I had later made me ill. In this case, this gym experience was nothing but misery, and chances are I wouldn't be eager to do it again anytime soon. When you start training for fun rather than just health, it becomes much easier.

The second big mistake that people make with the reward system is giving *large rewards for small efforts*. This is typical of people who believe that a couple of hours of playing sports is a great excuse to guzzle a case of beer. Another example is dieters who think that eating salad all week entitles them to eat a whole chocolate cake or go on a shopping spree that they can't really afford. Or the guy who makes a big production out of eating a few carrot sticks for supper and then heads out to the bar to knock back a few pitchers of beer because he "earned it."

The problem with large rewards for small efforts is that over time, you will need increasingly larger rewards to get the same result. Some dog trainers have this problem when they only use food as a reward. The dog will eventually only respond when it is hungry. It's also like bribing a spoiled child to do anything. The rewards have to get larger and larger to be effective.

The solution to this problem is to give *consistent, small rewards for regular efforts*. So, in the case of exercising, the trainee should follow up the exercise session with small rewards like watching a favorite show, telephoning a friend, or having a drink of juice. After a workout at a gym, one can schedule a walk through the mall or bookstore, a stop at a coffee shop, or whatever is routine and fun. One does not have to break the bank as part of a reward system.

The same goes for following an eating plan. By arranging the food to taste good or to take place in a good-time environment, you develop a mental link between eating healthy and enjoyment. For instance, there is probably not much fun to be had sitting at home alone and eating a low-calorie frozen meal. However, if you eat that same meal at a park, during a good television movie, or in good company, the meal becomes a pleasant experience. Personally, I would rather eat a hot dog in a park with friends than indulge in a gourmet meal at a high-class restaurant with company that I don't enjoy.

This method of small, consistent rewards can be applied to any regular task that you find challenging. It helped me immensely with my studies at university. As a reward for studying 15 extra minutes twice a day while traveling on the bus, I would get to read fiction for a designated period of time after each study session. Within a couple of months, I raised my Biology marks from a D to a B average.

Take the time to plan out your own small reward system to support your training program. A little bit of planning done now will pay off with big dividends later. See the behavior contract in Appendix C.

Behavior Modification Through Punishment

Obviously, if cigarettes tasted bad or booze caused instant hangovers, there would be fewer people smoking and drinking. Punishment for bad behavior is effective, but it has its limitations. First of all, the punishment has to be immediate; otherwise, there is no link between the punishment and the activity. For instance, if a dog owner beats a dog for something that the dog chewed up yesterday, the dog gets confused because it doesn't really understand what it is being punished for. The same goes for beating yourself up emotionally after missing exercise or eating too many desserts. The bad feelings (or punishment) that you have after the fact don't really link pain to the undesired action.

One way of teaching the mind negative consequences is through *avoidance conditioning.*[23] This is accomplished by causing some kind of mild pain during the unwanted activity. I tried this with a friend of mine who wanted to quit smoking. To help him quit, I got my friend to do 20 push-ups before every cigarette he smoked. This got him pumping out push-ups during every work break before he could have a cigarette. While it didn't get him to quit immediately, it did help get him into better physical condition, and as the days wore on, he found more and more excuses NOT to smoke. Six months later, he did finally give up smoking. And although he quit under his own willpower, he commented that the push-up routine really had helped.

I also knew a Pilates instructor who used to mark down on her cigarette package the number of cigarettes that she smoked throughout the day. At the end of the day, she would do several push-ups for every cigarette smoked. When I was trying to break a bad habit, I would do 50 or more push-ups before I did the activity (like eating junk food). After a few times of this routine, I found excuses not to do the activity.

Token System

Using a token system or token economy[24] is a variation of the reward system. Some of you may be familiar with the token systems used in schools (gold stars, letter grades), by credit card companies (air miles, reward points), auto insurance companies (demerit points for bad driving or discounts for good driving), and juvenile detention centers (points given or taken away based on behavior). And chances are that pretty much every one of you is familiar with the most universal of token systems…it's called money.

To use a token system, simply "pay" yourself a token every time you perform a desired action, like physical activity or eating properly. While any kind of token can be used, I prefer to pay myself money. This way, the reward is more tangible and immediate. For instance, for every hour of studying a difficult subject or writing that I do, I pay myself a dollar an hour. I also mark it on the calendar. Then, every weekend, I use the money to pay for some type of entertainment such as a movie, book, or going out to a restaurant. Keep in mind that like the reward system, the token must be spent soon and on something enjoyable. The amount really doesn't matter as much as the gesture. (Some people will pay themselves less than a dollar a day, while others can afford to pay themselves $50 a day.) However, saving up over several months or using the money for something necessary like car repairs or a telephone bill defeats the purpose of the reward. If all you can earn for yourself is $1.50, then make sure that you spend it on something or "toward" something that will feel like a treat.

The token system can also be used as a punishment, just like with traffic tickets. For instance, every time you eat junk food or skip a workout or activity session, you can give yourself a small fine. This can be a small amount of money (like a quarter) subtracted out of your reward system or a donation toward a charity. If you are competitive, you can make a pact with a friend to pay your fines to each other or pay the other's lunch at the end of the week.

One popular example of a *token system* of punishment is the decades-old "cuss box." With the cuss box, whenever someone swears (cusses), they have to pay a prescribed fine, dropping the appropriate amount into the cuss box. I used this method very successfully one summer as a "sarcasm box," after a co-worker remarked that certain sarcastic remarks were coming from my end of the office. To curb this habit, I would pay the sarcasm box between ten and twenty-five cents for every sarcastic remark that I made. This helped me stifle making certain remarks...for about a week. Then, as is common with many behavior changes, I had a relapse. In fact, there was such an intense return of my sarcasm habit that I just dropped five dollars into the box and let loose a week's worth of comments. After that, the habit simply faded. At the end of the month, I used the money in the box to take my co-worker out for food and drinks.

Although it is helpful to get started on new habits, eventually, you will want to wean yourself off the token system. There are two effective methods. The first method is to demand greater performance (like Frank running a quarter mile instead of walking around the house) for the same number of tokens. The second method is to increase the length of delay before the token is issued. This could mean that you give yourself a token at the end of the day or week for good performance. Personally, I keep using the token system on an ongoing basis for a few habits that are just plain hard to change. If a system works for you, use it.

Establishing a Routine

Ever notice how some people always have a cigarette with their coffee or drink? This is because an action performed with a routine activity will tend to reoccur with that routine activity. Often called the *Premack Principle,* it means developing a habit by coupling an uncommon activity like memorizing notes on a bathroom mirror with a common activity like shaving. If done frequently enough, the person shaving will tend to start looking for study notes whenever they get to a mirror for shaving.

To apply this to our exercise routines, we want to link a regular activity with physical activity. This can be something as simple as stretching while watching television or doing push-ups and crunches during commercial breaks. I once asked a very muscular 65-year-old martial arts instructor how he stayed in such good shape. He answered that he exercised lots and ate lots, usually while watching television. He mentioned that once he had performed 1,000 leg raises in front of the television set.

An even simpler method is to think positive thoughts during routine activities. This could include reciting a short pep talk every time you sit down for a meal or get behind the steering wheel of your car. One psychologist had his 17-year-old college student client imagine positive thoughts just before a trip to the urinal.[25] By coupling the two activities, the student automatically gave himself positive thoughts every time he went to the urinal (hopefully, the process did not reverse and make the guy lose bladder control every time he had a good thought).

In applying the *Premack Principle,* try to combine a desired behavior with your own normal routine. This might mean doing five or ten squats before and after shaving or doing the drawing-in-the-abdomen exercise every time you get in your automobile.

Delaying Gratification

In the military, we are taught the tactic of delaying the enemy at every opportunity. This strategy also works well for fighting bad habits, with the idea being that you *delay* the reward system or positive reinforcement involved with the bad habit. For instance, the simple technique of not having junk food in your home will force you to travel for it if you really want it. Another way to cut down on unwanted snacking is to put the snacks in a difficult place, like the attic or a high cupboard, to again *delay the gratification*. Some people who have difficulty with impulse buying freeze their credit cards in a block of ice so that they have to wait for the ice to melt to make their next purchase. *Delay, delay, delay...*

When it comes to delayed gratification, even subtle activities will work. For example, you can reduce overeating at the dinner table by putting down your utensils between bites. Aside from delaying the good taste of another mouthful of food, this can actually make you feel fuller with less food. Eating slower gives the body time to produce enough of the CCK (cholecystokinin) hormone to give you that feeling of fullness.

If you have couch-potato syndrome, you can delay the process of coming home and going straight for the living room couch. Some people avoid slacking off by making sure that they go directly to a gym after work. Others take their children for a walk or bike ride *as soon as they arrive home*. Find a suitable delay tactic and then make it part of your routine.

If you like dessert after supper, try to further delay it by having it *after* you wash the dishes or take out the garbage. Friends of mine insist that their children clean the supper dishes and do other chores *before* eating dessert. This not only delays the reward of eating dessert, but it also provides an incentive to complete certain chores that might otherwise be put off and gives you a greater sense of control.

No one ever said that delaying an unproductive (yet very enticing) course of action is easy. For instance, I once had the dilemma of stopping for a few cold beers after work or riding home on a hot, crowded bus. As I recall, it was a sweltering prairie day and I had been replacing toilets in an apartment complex for eight hours straight. On my way to the bus stop after work, I stepped into a bar to make a telephone call. The air inside the bar was cool and filled with the sound of clinking beer glasses, music, and friendly conversation. As I turned around after my call, I was faced with a difficult choice. Should I relax with a couple of cold brews until rush hour was over or step back outside into the wall of heat and board a stuffy, overcrowded bus? (Did I mention that I really hated riding that Friday afternoon bus?) Fortunately, for me, I had some goals to help pull me through. At the time, I was saving up money for university, and I also had plans to go out that evening. As it turned out, those two thoughts provided just enough incentive to drag me away from the inviting bar and onto that cattle car they called a bus for the ride home.

To overcome moments of weakness, plan ahead and have some kind of reward (or punishment) system already in place *before* you get sidetracked.

Environment

Planned environments, also known as *situational inducements,* can encourage certain behaviors. Grocery stores use bright displays and music to induce shoppers to buy more than they might have planned to. Fast-food restaurants use small, uncomfortable chairs to encourage patrons to eat and leave quickly.

During military parachute training at the Canadian Airborne Center, we were immersed in a physical training environment. Everywhere you looked, there was training equipment, chin-up bars, and motivational signs like "Try more push-ups" and "Do more chin-ups." Of course, the instructors were always nearby to provide encouragement (by yelling or commanding us to do push-ups or the "dry land" swim). We also had to run everywhere we went and shout the word "Airborne."

On the American base in Fort Bragg, North Carolina, I remember there were "monkey bars" in front of the mess (meal) halls. The trainees had to climb hand-over-hand along a sort of horizontal ladder as part of the meal lineup. Those who slipped and fell had to go back to the end of the lineup. The bottom line was that trainees either got a stronger grip or went hungry.

Following are four basic methods[26] that you can use to set up your own action environment to improve your fitness and overall health:

1. Rearrange Your Surroundings

Rearranging your surroundings provides several options. If you respond best to visual stimulus, you can put up motivational quotes, written reminders, or pictures of athletes that inspire you. If what you need is a motivational nudge, you can move your bed near a window to catch the morning sun or put an exercise mat in the middle of your living room so that it is the first thing you see when you come home. I usually keep a gym bag full of workout gear by the front door as a reminder.

2. Find a New Location

The old saying, "A change is as good as a rest" is true for most people, and just having something different to look at while you work out can be refreshing. If you've been working out at home or in the office, try a new location such as a park, gym, community center, or training area. For most people, it is far easier to train in a place where exercise is the norm; this will likely help to boost your motivation.

3. Relocate People

Relocating people is about keeping the right company for certain situations, like physical activity. Training buddies can help keep each other motivated (or drag each other down). Try to train and talk with fitness-oriented people and avoid less-motivated people. It is hard enough changing your habits without hearing snide remarks from other people. Be very selective who you share your goals with.

4. Change the Time of the Activity

Optimizing the time of day that you engage in an activity can be helpful for both physical training and weight control. Some people have higher energy levels first thing in the morning—or at midday— than they do later on. If this is you, take full advantage of timing to schedule your activities. I used to teach a Pilates fitness class during lunch hour and then eat a light lunch at my desk before carrying on with my work. I found that I got more done this way and stayed more alert during the day than I had previously when I stayed at my desk and ate a large lunch in one sitting. Speaking of eating, sometimes cooking the next day's meal right *after* you eat your evening meal can help prevent overeating. This way, because you are already full, there is less of a tendency to nibble and sample the meal during cooking.

The key to making the environmental approach work is being aware of how different elements in your surroundings affect you. If you haven't already, make a list of all of the positive people, places, times, and opportunities for exercise and eating right. Work at making these situations happen. Next, make a list of all of the negative people, places, times, and events that influence inactivity and poor health habits, then work at avoiding these situations. Above all, keep negative behaviors away from your new environments (e.g., smoking or eating junk food at a gym). Like a military operation, use every situation to your advantage.

Relapses

A good plan always takes into account the human tendency to slide back into old habits. Unfortunately, when it happens, many people have a tendency to beat themselves up over missing a workout or try to catch up by doing multiple workouts or starving themselves as punishment. You need to expect—and learn to accept—the occasional setback in any diet or training program. This is why it is important to plan ahead to prevent "falling off of the wagon."

Let's look at some typical scenarios:

Avoidable Situations

If you know your weaknesses, certain places can be avoided. For example, if pastries are your downfall, rather than frequenting a coffee shop that sells pastries, you can choose to go to one that doesn't. Or at least avoid that coffee shop during the first month of your program when your new habits are forming.

Unavoidable Situations

If due to business or other commitments, you cannot avoid a place like the coffee shop that sells pastries, you can always bring the exact change needed for your tea or coffee or choose to sit with your back to the display case.

Overreaction to Occasional Setbacks

There is something about human nature that strives to keep things the same. I have yet to meet even one person who has *never* had a relapse back into a bad habit. Even the most disciplined people will miss a week of workouts, eat two dozen muffins in a day, or go on a week of partying. I get small relapses all the time. It is not a big deal *unless you make it a big deal.* When you do have a setback, instead of beating yourself up emotionally, take the time to review all the times that you stayed with the program. Then get back on the wagon and keep moving forward.

Counterproductive Self-Talk

Counterproductive self-talk is what I like to call a "what's the use" attitude. Here are some examples: "I'm never going to be a super athlete, so why should I bother exercising at all?" or "Everyone else is way ahead of me/better than me, so what's the point?" It is important to recognize this kind of behavior for what it is: your mind's knee-jerk response to fatigue. Remind yourself that fatigue is just a temporary condition and as your body gets stronger, this little voice will eventually disappear.

Too Much Too Soon

Trying to do too much too soon is one of the most common reasons for the failure of a new fitness program. I know two different people who have attempted to run a full marathon after just a few weeks of mild training, with no previous experience. As a youth, I recall that I was constantly trying to imitate advanced strength-building routines without using the proper technique or incorporating the necessary elements of rest and nutrition into my regimen. Over the years, I have seen hundreds of poorly conditioned people at various gyms push themselves beyond their fitness level for a couple of weeks and then disappear. As the saying goes, eat your elephant one bite at a time. Progress, not perfection is the goal.

Too Much of a Good Thing

Over-training is a common problem with many fitness enthusiasts. The symptoms of over-training include: an accelerated heart rate, sleeplessness, tendency to be injury-prone, fatigue, and staleness. Unfortunately, some of us get a bit of a high from over-training and find it difficult to stop exercising. If you think that you are burning out, try a couple of light days of training or change up your routines. You will often find that you come back even stronger than before. Keep in mind that while exercise is an important part of a healthy lifestyle, you must remember to eat, rest, and sleep as well.

Planning Isn't About Being Perfect

I used to skip planning with the belief that it was taking up valuable training time. Whereas a cyclist friend of mine made meticulous training plans. Every workout, he knew exactly what he wanted to improve. I began to take notice when he surpassed me in skill and strength training within a short period. After that, I found that my progress was far better when I at least had some kind of plan to follow. The danger with some plans is that they can lead you into that popular all-or-nothing kind of attitude. Some perfectionists will refuse to train unless it is for a full hour in their favorite gym or only with certain equipment. Since time, equipment, food, and rest are not always going to fit your schedule, you have to make adjustments occasionally for typical disruptions. For instance, if you've had to work late and not yet had supper, you can still eat a light supper, do some of your exercises, and then eat the rest of your supper later. You cannot expect to have perfect workouts, meals, etc. every time. Some training is better than none. Again, think progress, not perfection.

Chapter 8
Overcoming Flat Gut Roadblocks

A Beer Gut Case Study

Before I reveal what finally worked, let's examine what the typical beer gut consists of. First, there is a layer of cutaneous fat just under the skin that accumulates around the midriff. Next, there is visceral fat that collects around the intestines. Finally, the gut itself hangs because of a few things:

1. Displaced internal organs. The internal organs belong inside the protective cage of the ribs. The bloated gut makes them hang out of place. This can be corrected with breathing and exercise.

2. A bloated colon. Some people's large intestines are so full of waste that the colon itself bulges. Not good for health or appearance.

3. Pelvic tilt. A warped posture too tight of hamstrings and lower back will cause the pelvis to tilt forward and let the stomach hang and butt stick out. This is unhealthy and puts extra strain on the lower back.

4. Cortisol. Stress can produce cortisol, which can disrupt sleep and cause weight gain.

Without losing an ounce, the right exercises can align the body and *draw the gut* back inside the rib cage (where it is supposed to be). If you do not believe me, squeeze your shoulder blades together and observe how your chest goes out and your abdomen is drawn in.

The right food will not only reduce the layer of fat on someone's body, it will also keep the colon clean and healthy and remove the excess waste.

And believe it or not, reducing stress by eating, sleeping, and training *moderately* was more effective than over-training. In the case of my client, he lost the most size and weight around his beer gut when he took a few days off of training (and following my advice). With his lower cortisol levels, his body was able to build more muscle and burn more fat.

Putting It All Together

Ultimately, your stomach-flattening workouts will give you increased strength and energy—if you apply them. Despite distractions and interruptions related to family, career, education, accidents, or even the occasional natural disaster, there is always going to be some way of overcoming your obstacles.

I hope that you enjoyed Flat Gut After 50. If you would like to receive more information on books, courses, and information, I will put you on my VIP mailing list. We would love to hear of your success. Go to www.2ndwindbodyscience.com.

ABOUT THE AUTHOR

Doug Setter is a former paratrooper, United Nations peace-keeper, and champion kickboxer. He is the author of *Strength Endurance Secrets, Reduce Your Alcohol Craving, Simple Secrets to Handle Your Alcohol Better: Student's Edition, One Less Victim,* and award winner youth literature novel, *Selo.*

He works and lives in Vancouver, Canada and can be reached through his website: www.2ndwindbodyscience.com

APPENDIX A:
METABOLIC TYPE TEST
(Based on The Balance by Oz Garcia)

1. Do you tend to get angry?
    a. Easily
    b. Almost never
    c. Occasionally

2. Do you tend to get anxious?
    a. Easily
    b. Almost never
    c. Occasionally

3. Your appetite is:
    a. Above normal
    b. Below normal
    b. Normal

4. You find it easy to:
    a. Lose weight
    b. Gain weight
    c. Maintain weight

5. Your hair is usually:
    a. Dry
    b. Oily
    c. Normal

6. Your skin is usually:
    a. Dry
    b. Oily
    c. Normal

7. Bedtime eating makes you:
    a. Toss and turn all night
    b. Feel good
    c. Indifferent

8. During the day, you:
    a. Sometimes forget to eat
    b. Get hungry often
    c. Eat only 3 times per day

9. Emotionally, you tend toward:
    a. A hot temper
    b. Calm, cool, and collected
    c. Occasional emotional upsets

10. You exercise:
    a. Frequently and enjoy it
    b. Seldom, and dislike it
    c. Sometimes and enjoy it

11. You fall asleep:
    a. Easily
    b. With difficulty
    c. Within half an hour

12. You feel fatigue:
    a. Seldom
    b. Often
    c. Occasionally

13. If exercising, you like to choose:
    a. Intense aerobic exercise
    b. Weights and machines
    c. Either or

14. Your blood sugar is usually
    a. Low
    b. High
    c. Normal

15. Your breakfast is usually:
    a. Skipped
    b. Large
    c. Average

16. You like raw salad and vegetables:
    a. Quite a bit
    b. Indifferent
    c. Sometimes

17. You tend to feel too warm:
    a. Very rarely
    b. Frequently
    c. Rarely

18. You are most alert:
    a. Bright and early
    b. Around noon
    c. Whenever you get up

19. Around evening, you tend to:
    a. Go to bed early
    b. Come alive
    c. Gradually slow down

20. Regardless of what you eat, you:
    a. Have trouble gaining weight
    b. Gain weight easily
    c. Have stable weight

21. Your stamina is:
    a. Above normal
    b. Low
    c. Normal

Total the letters. As = Fast Burners, Bs = Slow Burners, Cs = Mixed Burners

APPENDIX B:
WORKOUT JOURNAL

Starting weight _____

Measurements _____

Month _____

Sun	Mon	Tue	Wed	Thur	Fri	Sat
work out, eat, rest						

Total number of workouts _____ /30 days

DIET: B = Bad, OK = Okay, G = Good

APPENDIX C:
BEHAVIOR-CHANGING CONTRACT

LIFESTYLE CONTRACT

Designed by Doug Setter

1. My specific goals for lifestyle change are:

   _____

2. Short-term self-control goals are:

   _____

3. I will journal my progress every _____ and review in ____ days
   on the date of:

4. To minimize the causes of the problem, I will:

   _____

5. Rewards for short-term goals:

   _____

6. Minor punishments for straying from a program:
   (e.g., no music for a day)

   _____

7. Additional steps for success:

   _____

(Date)

(Your Signature)

(Supporter's Signature)

REFERENCES

1. Borugian, M.J, Sheps, S.B, Kim-Sing, C, Olivotto, I.A., Van Patten, C, Dunn, B.P., Coldman, A.J., Potter, J.D., Gallagher, R.P. & Hislop, T.G. (2003) Am. J. Epdemiol Nov. 158:963-968. . . . . Note: High insulin levels have been associated with increased risk of breast cancer and poorer survival after a breast cancer diagnosis. Waist-to-hip ratio (WHR) is a marker for insulin resistance and hyperinsulinemia.

2. An abdominal crunch is performed by lying on your back and curling your upper body forward so that the shoulder blades are off the ground.

3. Yesudian, Selvarajan and Haich, Elisabeth (1953) Yoga and Health. Harper and Row Publishers: New York.

4. Ibid. p.117.

5. Christensen, Alice (1995) 20-Minute Yoga Workouts. Ballantine Books: New York.

6. Null, Gary, PhD (1999) Gary Null's Ultimate Anti-Aging Program. p. 297-298.

7. Stefansson, V (1964) Discovery: The Autobiography of Vilhjalmur Stefansson McGraw-Hill: New York. 1964.

8. Kirschmann, John D. with Dunne, Lavon J. (1984) Nutrition Almanac. McGraw-Hill: New York.

9. Fredericks, Carlton, Ph.D. (1988) Psycho-Nutrition. Berkley Books: New York.

10. Ibid.

11. Pearson, Durk and Shaw, Sandy (1983) Life Extension: A Practical Scientific Approach. Warner Books, Inc.:New York. P.370.

12. Mathews-Larson (1997) 7 Weeks to Sobriety. Ballantine Books: New York.

13. Fredericks, Carlton, Ph.D. (1988) Psycho-Nutrition. Berkley Books: New York.

14. Garcia, Oz w/Kolberg, Sharyn (1998) The Balance. Regan Books: New York. P.19.

15. Ibid.

16. Banting, William (1864) On Corpulence, Harrison: London.

17. A friend of mine fell susceptible to a blood disease after fasting for several months. From his weakened state, a former blood disease re-emerged and he died. Fasting can have its own mild high and should be treated cautiously.

18. Mackarness, Richard (1976) Not All in the Mind. Pan Books Ltd.: London.

19. Gordon, J (2007) https://www.pnas.org/content/101/44/15718

20. Gawain, Shakti (1978) Creative Visualization. Bantam Books: New York. P. 80-84.

21. Martin, Garry, Pear, Joseph (1999) Behavior Modification: What it is and How to do it. Prentice Hall P.27.

22. Ibid.

23. Ibid. p.177-178.

24. Ibid.

25. Ibid.

26. Ibid.

Made in the USA
Las Vegas, NV
28 February 2022

44714891R00069